T0200200

DSM-5® POCKET GUIDE for
Elder Mental Health

DSM-5® POCKET GUIDE for
Elder Mental Health

Sophia Wang, M.D.

Medical Director, Older Adult Mental Health Clinic, Richard L. Roudebush VA Medical Center
Assistant Clinical Professor, Indiana University School of Medicine
Implementation Scientist, Center for Health Innovation and Implementation Science
Physician, Eskenazi Healthy Aging Brain, Indianapolis, Indiana

Abraham M. Nussbaum, M.D., FAPA

Chief Education Officer, Denver Health
Associate Professor, Department of Psychiatry, University of Colorado School of Medicine, Denver, Colorado

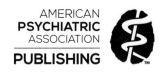

AMERICAN
PSYCHIATRIC
ASSOCIATION
PUBLISHING

Copyright © 2017 American Psychiatric Association Publishing

ALL RIGHTS RESERVED

First Edition

Manufactured in the United States of America on acid-free paper

20   19   18   17   16   5   4   3   2   1

American Psychiatric Association Publishing

1000 Wilson Boulevard

Arlington, VA 22209-3901

www.appi.org

Library of Congress Cataloging-in-Publication Data

Names: Wang, Sophia, 1979– author. | Nussbaum, Abraham M., 1975– author. | American Psychiatric Association, issuing body.

Title: DSM-5 pocket guide for elder mental health / Sophia Wang, Abraham M. Nussbaum.

Other titles: Pocket guide for elder mental health | Diagnostic and statistical manual of mental disorders-5 pocket guide for elder mental health | Diagnostic and statistical manual of mental disorders-five pocket guide for elder mental health

Description: First edition. | Arlington, Virginia : American Psychiatric Association Publishing, [2017] | Includes bibliographical references and index.

Identifiers: LCCN 2016036552 (print) | LCCN 2016037168 (ebook) | ISBN 9781615370566 (pb : alk. paper) | ISBN 9781615371198 (ebook)

Subjects: | MESH: Diagnostic and statistical manual of mental disorders. 5th ed. | Mental Disorders—diagnosis | Aged | Mental Disorders—therapy | Interview, Psychological—methods | Handbooks

Classification: LCC RC469 (print) | LCC RC469 (ebook) | NLM WT 39 | DDC 616.89/075--dc23

LC record available at https://lccn.loc.gov/2016036552

British Library Cataloguing in Publication Data A CIP record is available from the British Library.

Contents

SECTION I
Diagnosing and Treating Older Adults

SECTION II
Using DSM-5 With Older Adults

SECTION III
Additional Tools and Initial Treatments

Preface

The release of DSM-5 (American Psychiatric Association 2013) renewed public interest in how to evaluate a person in distress for the presence of a mental illness (e.g., American Psychiatric Association 2015b; American Psychiatric Association Work Group on Psychiatric Evaluation 2016; Moseley and Gala 2015). For most observers, the core issue was how to distinguish variants of normal behavior from pathological states. When the use of DSM-5 with older adults was initially debated, the discussion focused on whether or not the removal of the bereavement exemption from the diagnosis of major depressive disorder turned grief into a pathological state.

The question of whether an older adult's experience is best described as depression or grieving opens a broader debate about the boundaries between mental illness and normal age-related changes. For example, you may have to decide whether an elder is experiencing depression or grief, a sleep disorder or age-related insomnia, or a neurocognitive disorder or the memory losses attendant on aging. A determination as to whether an older person is experiencing a mental illness or an age-related process is never simple, because it involves many aspects of an individual's life, including culture, ethnicity, faith, family history, gender, medical history, sexual orientation, social history, and temperament. A thorough evaluation typically includes an extended history; an account of the individual's current and future needs for support; his or her chronological age and functional age; the temperament of the individual and his or her caregivers; and the health of both the person and his or her family. In short, you have to get to know another person. We believe DSM-5 is a way to begin this kind of evaluation, this way of knowing.

The way is not, however, straightforward. For example, DSM-5 is a manual for the diagnosis of mental illness in a particular person. Using it with older adults, whose health is inevitably bound up in their communities and families, requires an act of translation. Similarly, this book is a translation of DSM-5. It is not a replacement for DSM-5 itself or for the many psychiatric textbooks now available for the care of older adults (e.g., Steffens et al. 2015; Thakur et al. 2013), but rather presents a way to employ DSM-5 criteria as part of a person-centered interview and an evidence-based treatment plan.

We have written this book for practitioners at all levels of experience, including students, trainees, and fellow practitioners. The first section introduces the diagnostic interview, its goals, and how to structure an interview based on how much time you have with a person. The second section operationalizes the DSM-5 diagnostic criteria for clinical practice. The third section includes additional information, tables, and tools for initiating a treatment plan. Taken as a whole, this book helps you accurately diagnose and treat an older adult in mental distress while establishing a therapeutic alliance.

Before we begin, we have a few comments about language used in this book. When possible, we use neutral gender for the person and the interviewer, but when doing so is grammatically awkward, we alternate between the universal feminine in odd-numbered chapters and the universal masculine in even-numbered chapters.

To emphasize an older adult's agency—his or her ability to act in the world—we use the word *person* to describe the object of mental health evaluation. A robust debate exists about whether the object of medical care is best construed as an ill patient under the care of a health professional or as an autonomous consumer of that professional's services (see Emanuel and Emanuel 1992; Mol 2008; Tomes 2016), but because personhood precedes illness or consumption, we prefer to use the word *person*. However, when we write about someone who has entered psychiatric treatment, we use the term *patient* because this word acknowledges both the vulnerability of the person in treatment and the responsibilities assumed by professionals when they care for patients (Radden and Sadler 2010). We use the term *patient* not to endorse medical paternalism but to emphasize that the particular and protected relationships that develop in clinical encounters are better described as therapeutic relationships than as therapeutic contracts.

Because older adults often depend on a variety of others—spouses, siblings, children, extended family members, friends, faith leaders, neighbors, coworkers, and more—for their needs, we use the term *caregiver* to describe someone who helps an older adult seek health outside of a medical relationship.

Older adults receive care within medical relationships from persons trained in a variety of helping professions. To acknowledge this variety, we use the term *practitioner* to describe a health professional who cares for older adults. Although *provider* is the more common euphemism, we prefer *practitioner* because it emphasizes the ways a professional who meets older adults as patients is constantly practicing and refining his or her craft.

Finally, we are both early in our careers as physicians and still have much to learn, both with and from the people we meet as our patients. Using the term *elder* to describe our older patients emphasizes both the difference in age and the difference in experience between our patients and us. We learn from our elders, even as we care for them.

Acknowledgments

We thank the professional elders who have shared their wisdom with us—Dan Blazer, Malaz Boustani, Nancy Clayton, Vince Collins, Mary DeMay, Hillel Grossman, Helen Hoenig, Craig Holland, Robert House, Barbara Kamholz, Thomas McAllister, Bruce Miller, Arnaldo Moreno, Craig Nelson, Judith Neugroschl, Mary Sano, Lea Watson, Joel Yager, and Kristine Yaffe—and our respective institutions for supporting this endeavor. We thank Libby Davies, who read and improved an early draft, and the editorial staff at American Psychiatric Association Publishing for their careful attention. Finally, we thank our patients; our patients' caregivers; and our families, especially the older adults in our personal lives, who inspired this book.

Disclosures

Abraham M. Nussbaum, M.D., FAPA, reports royalties from Yale University Press.
Sophia Wang, M.D., reports no conflicting interests.

SECTION I

Diagnosing and Treating
Older Adults

CHAPTER 1

Introduction

After a lifetime of seeking medical assistance only for emergencies, Pat, a 67-year-old woman, is belatedly establishing a primary care relationship at the request of her adult daughter Kate. Pat was recently hospitalized for an unintentional overdose of pain medications; while going through her mother's home, Kate discovered that Pat was taking five different types of pain pills from four different doctors. Kate, who has accompanied her mother, wants you to help organize Pat's care.

Kate tells you that a few years ago a neurologist diagnosed Pat with "mild memory problems." Over the past year, she has had increasing trouble finding words and answering questions meaningfully. Pat is fairly independent—she can drive to familiar places, cook simple meals, and run errands without difficulty—but needs help when driving to new places and, as Kate has discovered, when taking medications.

Kate tells you all this before Pat says anything. When you ask Pat how she is doing and what today's date is, she replies, "I'm fine." She says nothing else. When you repeat your question about today's date, Pat responds, "My daughter knows everything else. Why don't you ask her what day it is." While Pat glares at the wall, Kate starts to cry.

You feel frustrated as you open up Pat's electronic health record. It includes a screen-long problem list, each problem associated with a medication or two, and 6 years' worth of notes from her neurologist and three other subspecialists, who apparently have never communicated with each other. You have 15 minutes to organize this information, assess Pat's mental health, reassure her daughter, and stifle your own feelings of being overwhelmed.

We too have felt overwhelmed when caring for older adults with uncharacterized needs who are receiving uncoordinated care. After many years, we learned to transform our frustrations into effective strategies; we offer this guide to share the lessons we have learned from our mentors and from our own experiences. We provide accessible strategies for assessing and addressing the mental health needs of older adults.

What Is in This Book

Many practitioners fear treating mental health issues in older people because of beliefs that special expertise is required; however, we believe that all practitioners can learn to feel confident about working with older people. Our goal is to help you build confidence in your ability to care for older patients with mental health needs and to nurture your interest in working with the people who make up this rapidly growing segment of the population. We describe how to perform a brief interview, recognize the main elements of the most common mental health disorders, reach an initial diagnosis, engage patients in treatment, work with other caregivers, and, if necessary, know when to refer patients for additional subspecialty mental health treatment.

Gaining confidence in caring for older patients comes from building relationships with them and their caregivers. Relationships develop through stories. To model this, we share stories drawn from our clinical experience so you can learn the following essential skills:

- Recognizing that the same chief complaint can result in different diagnoses (Chapter 3)
- Performing a 15- or 30-minute version of a diagnostic interview when you are considering different diagnostic possibilities (Chapters 5 and 6)
- Measuring and following the symptoms of a patient's mental illness and psychosocial functioning (Chapters 10 and 11) as you decide between diagnoses
- Initiating psychosocial (Chapter 14), psychotherapeutic (Chapter 15), psychopharmacological (Chapter 16) treatment, and brain stimulation interventions (Chapter 17) once you have arrived at the best diagnosis

Each chapter focuses on the most common mental health disorders in older adults. We hope practitioners working outside behavioral health clinics and hospitals will grow confident in diagnosing and managing these disorders. To aid you, we have designed this book with easy-to-use tips, tables, and treatment guidelines tied to the DSM-5 diagnostic criteria sets (American Psychiatric Association 2013). We developed these diagnostic and treatment aids after working in various clinical roles, including consulting psychiatrist to geriatric medicine and primary care services, outpatient adult psychiatrist in an intake clinic, psychotherapist for adults struggling with aging, emergency psychiatrist, and inpatient psychiatrist. We have provided both psychotherapy and medication treatments for older people. We include a range of treatments because we understand that the way geriatric mental health conditions are treated varies widely by setting and access to mental health and social services. Despite our many years of working with older adults, we continue to be surprised by what we learn from our patients and their caregivers and still frequently consult colleagues and brainstorm new ideas for treatment. We remain humble each time we meet a new elder as a patient and are always eager to learn from her, her caregivers, and her other practitioners.

The definition of *older adult* has changed over the years. In the past, geriatric care was initiated when a patient turned 60 or 65. Today, we prefer to initiate a geriatric approach to medical care when it suits the patient. We determine whether an adult is functionally geriatric by considering the severity of medical and mental illness and functional status alongside her chronological age. A 55-year-old patient with progressive dementia secondary to severe traumatic brain injury would benefit from the approaches described in this guide and, if available, geriatric subspecialty care. In contrast, a primary care practitioner may care for a fairly healthy 75-year-old with mild depressive symptoms who functions independently.

Four Concepts That Define Geriatric Psychiatry

1. **Everyone has a story.** We learn individual life stories from our patients and their caregivers, so we need to take the time to bond, laugh, and cry with them.
2. **Treatment must have functional benefit.** We do not recommend tests or treatments that offer no benefit to a patient. We would not, for example, prescribe donepezil for a 95-year-old woman who has end-stage dementia resulting in poor functional status, even though the U.S. Food

and Drug Administration has approved donepezil for dementia.

3. **Practitioners care for both the patient and her caregivers.** As a patient functionally declines, she increasingly relies on caregivers to make appointments and follow treatment regimens. Therefore, if a caregiver is not implementing treatment recommendations, we work to ensure implementation or initiate other resources if she is having difficulty.

4. **Simple works best.** We try to stop unnecessary medications before starting a new one. Similarly, we first introduce simple lifestyle changes such as asking our patients to walk 10 more minutes when they do their routine grocery shopping before we ask them to run a half-mile.

Behavioral and Mental Distress Seen in Older Adults

An older adult experiencing mental illness usually comes to a practitioner's attention when the patient, a caregiver, or the practitioner identifies a distressing behavioral or mental symptom. Common examples of behavioral distress include sleep problems, physical complaints that cannot be explained entirely by medical illness, social isolation, and substance use. Common examples of mental distress include excessive worry, enduring sadness, declining cognitive ability, thoughts of suicide, and suspiciousness of others. Less common examples of distress include perceptual disturbances such as auditory and visual hallucinations, compulsive behaviors, and even homicidal thoughts.

DIFFERENCES BETWEEN MENTAL DISTRESS AND MENTAL ILLNESS

Imagine that while seeing Pat for the first time, you tell her, "Kate seems very concerned about you." Pat replies, "I'm fine. I want to go home now." You encourage her to stay and complete the visit so you can ask screening questions about appetite, mood, and sleep. Pat agrees, but then she folds her arms over her chest and answers "fine" to all questions. Kate catches your eye and says, unbidden, "Mom's lost 10 pounds in the past 3 months. She watches TV in her bed all day and sleeps badly at night." You share Kate's concern that although Pat reports being fine, her memory symptoms have progressed from mental distress to mental illness.

Mental distress is often characterized by the 4 Ss: *self-resolution* of symptoms in a brief period of time (usually days to weeks), response to *short-term supportive* interventions alone (e.g., a couple of counseling sessions or a short-term support group), *self-awareness* of symptoms and their impact on functioning, and *stable functioning*. Usually, people with mental distress have no previous psychiatric history or recent psychiatric contact, no previous use of psychotropic medications, and a high level of functioning prior to the current episode.

Mental illness is usually characterized by the 4 Ps: the *progression* of symptoms if a person does not receive treatment, *persistence* and *poor awareness* of symptoms, and *poor functioning* due to these symptoms. Poor awareness of symptoms may be from anosognosia (a lack of awareness due to brain damage) and may indicate decreased motivation for successful participation in mental health treatment. A common example of anosognosia is a patient, like Pat, with major neurocognitive disorder who is not aware of her memory problem. An additional sign of mental illness may be that another person accompanies the patient to the visit, although patients who present alone may not be functioning independently. Although recurring symptoms suggest mental illness, neurocognitive disorders are distinct among the major mental illnesses because their first presentation usually occurs as an adult ages. If you cannot determine, after an initial interview, whether an older adult is experiencing distress or illness, you should explain that the diagnosis is not yet clear but that assistance is already available. You can follow a patient to see if her symptoms resolve on their own, initiate an intervention, and alter your approach as needed.

FREQUENCY OF BEHAVIORS AND MENTAL DISORDERS

In 2010, about 5.6–8 million older adults had a mental health or substance use disorder (Institute of Medicine 2012). The prevalence of these disorders, however, varies widely by setting. For example, delirium is usually diagnosed in a hospital rather than a community setting, making the prevalence in hospitals much higher. The higher the level of care a patient requires, the higher the overall prevalence of mental health disorders. In the United States, about 11% of older adults have Alzheimer's disease (the most common type of major neurocognitive disorder), whereas 30% of home health patients and nearly 50% of patients in a long-term-care facility have major neurocognitive disorder (Alzheimer's and other types) (Alzheimer's Association 2015a; Harris-Kojetin et al. 2016). Similarly, whereas less than 25% of patients in adult day service centers and residential care communities have depression, nearly half of all patients in long-term-care settings are depressed (Harris-Kojetin et al. 2013).

Among older adults who were living in the community, less than 6% reported having a depressive disorder (major depressive disorder or dysthymic disorder) or an anxiety disorder (panic disorder, social phobia, or generalized anxiety disorder) (Institute of Medicine 2012). About 2% reported having posttraumatic stress disorder or a substance use disorder, and less than 1% reported having bipolar disorder, schizophrenia, or obsessive-compulsive disorder (Institute of Medicine 2012).

USE OF A DIAGNOSTIC INTERVIEW TO DISTINGUISH BETWEEN MENTAL DISTRESS AND MENTAL ILLNESS

The gold standard for diagnosis of psychiatric disorders is the clinical interview; one of its major purposes is to distinguish between mental distress and mental illness. As you interview someone, remember the 4 Ss and 4 Ps. Specifically, ask about the *progression* and *persistence* of symptoms and the impairment of functioning secondary to these symptoms. Questions such as "How long has this been going on?" and "Have you had symptoms similar to this at any other time in your life?" can clarify whether you are dealing with a brief episode of the blues, a first depressive episode, or recurrent major depressive disorder. Assessing function is so essential to diagnosis and treatment that we discuss it in detail in Chapter 11. In brief, you should be sure to assess a patient's social functioning, instrumental activities of daily living, and activities of daily living. Finally, all practitioners should be alert to red flags for mental illness that may necessitate consultation with a general psychiatrist or, if possible, a geriatric psychiatrist (Table 1–1). In some cases, red flags may require referral to the emergency department for urgent assessment and psychiatric admission.

One commonly held belief is that the diagnostic interview is completed on the first visit. We believe that the diag-

TABLE 1–1. Red flags for mental illness

Previous inpatient psychiatric hospitalizations

High risk for suicide

Previous suicide attempts, especially those resulting in medical hospitalization

Ready access to firearms or other weapons and presence of mental health symptoms

Symptoms of mania or psychosis

Previous treatment with psychotropic medication, electroconvulsive therapy, or other neurostimulation treatments

nostic mental health interview is a tool to be used at every visit, just like a stethoscope. With the interview, you can assess a patient's well-being while reassessing the validity of a diagnosis. Although the strongest evidence for a correct diagnosis is usually a positive response to treatment, you should always remember that the relationship between treatment and improvement can be a coincidence. With each patient encounter, you should perform a portion of the diagnostic interview to collect additional information to confirm your diagnosis, add a diagnosis to your differential, or exclude a diagnosis. To avoid premature conclusions, you can repeat portions of the diagnostic interview as you learn more about a patient.

Therapeutic Alliance: The Key to Accurate Diagnosis and Successful Treatment

The therapeutic alliance is the relationship a practitioner and a patient form in pursuit of the patient's health or well-being. In a strong therapeutic alliance, both practitioner and patient feel a positive emotional connection and trust each other. In a weak alliance, the practitioner or the patient feels hostile toward the other, the patient frequently does not follow treatment recommendations, and the practitioner experiences frustration with the patient's noncompliance. A strong alliance can determine whether an older adult decides to seek mental health treatment or to suffer without it. It is especially necessary to develop a therapeutic alliance with patients who have internalized stigma toward anyone with mental illness before they can be successfully engaged in mental health treatment.

ALLIANCE BUILDING WITH AN OLDER PERSON

Consider the first visit with Pat. She was brought to treatment against her wishes and stayed only at your insistence. As the first visit comes to its merciful conclusion, you may feel demoralized. So may Kate; it took her weeks to convince her mother to see a psychiatrist, and Pat told you little more than that she is "fine" and does not need treatment. As you hand Pat a slip for a follow-up appointment, you doubt she will ever return.

After she walks away, you seek out a colleague for encouragement and counsel. Your colleague suggests, "Get to know Pat as a person. Don't ask her if she is depressed. Find out what she likes to do, and then ask whether she is still enjoying it."

When Pat surprises you by returning for a second visit, you decide to interview her alone and begin by asking, "What do you like to do for fun?" Pat replies, "I used to read and play tennis. But now I just watch travel shows on TV." You ask more about her interest in travel. Toward the end of the visit, Pat confides in you that she and Kate were estranged because Pat's second husband, Oscar, did not get along with Kate. They reconciled after Oscar died 2 years ago. Now Pat is very angry because she feels that Kate forced her to come to mental health treatment as a "punishment" for marrying Oscar against Kate's wishes. Pat agrees to return, at least so she can talk more about her frustrations with Kate.

As demonstrated in Pat's case, building a therapeutic alliance with older people often takes a few meetings. Changes in cognitive function and social circumstances lead many older adults to be cautious; they may need more time than do younger people to process information. Many older adults have never needed mental health treatment, so they may take longer to feel connected and comfortable with the idea of being a "psych patient." To proactively address their concerns, we usually spend a couple of minutes at the beginning of the appointment setting expectations. We explain the purpose of the visit (e.g., mental health referral for depression, part of mental health screening in primary care), the length of the appointment (e.g., 5 minutes for a screening vs. 30 or 60 minutes for a mental health visit), what the patient can hope to get out of the visit at the end, and the expected length of the relationship (one or multiple visits). Building a therapeutic alliance can also take several meetings because many older people feel as though they are being ignored by their own family and friends and wonder whether practitioners will ignore them as well. If you feel that a person is experiencing mental distress, even though she denies any symptoms, you may want to extend your initial assessment over two sessions. People who are depressed or lonely may open up only on a second visit, so you need enough of a therapeutic alliance that the second visit occurs.

> At Pat's third visit, you talk further about her feelings toward mental health treatment. Pat says, "Kate is punishing me by trying to drug me up." You reassure her by saying, "I can see you are concerned. Can we begin by talking about your experiences with mental health treatment?"
> Pat describes the pain of seeing her own mother endure multiple "shock treatments" for schizophrenia. In response, you educate her about today's mental health treatments: "Now, we often integrate mental health treatment into a primary care setting. For example, I am your primary care physician, and I care for both your physical and mental health needs. Mental health care is very different today than when your mother was treated. Most care takes place in the clinic, and we have a number of effective medications that people take by mouth. Most of my patients do well and live independently." By the end of the visit, Pat agrees to try a small dose of a selective serotonin reuptake inhibitor so she can have enough energy to get out of the house again.

Patients often express, directly or indirectly, an unwillingness to be evaluated for mental health problems, saying things like "I'm not crazy!" or "I don't believe in psychiatry." When we hear these kinds of comments, we do not take them personally but consider them as the place to start; when a person can verbalize her fears, she has offered an area for education. We build the therapeutic alliance by encouraging a wary person to verbalize her fears and by educating her on the realities of contemporary mental health treatment.

Some patients are both unwary and unaware. They present for initial evaluation as pleasant and cheerful, denying any problem, without expressing fear about mental health treatment or even the reason for referral. In this situation, we start by asking about the patient's daily routine, her hobbies and interests, and what she has seen recently on the news. The responses can give you a sense of the patient's functional performance and orientation while simultaneously giving the patient the opportunity to open up to you as a person. It is important to get details to make sure the information is up to date. A patient will sometimes minimize her symptoms by describing her functioning before mental health symptoms developed. For example, if a patient states that she is an avid reader, the practitioner could ask more detailed questions such as "When was the last time you read a book that you enjoyed? What was the book about? What books are you reading now?"

QUICK TIPS FOR BUILDING A THERAPEUTIC ALLIANCE WITH OLDER ADULTS

Address older adults by their last names with the proper titles (Dr., Mr., Mrs., Ms.) until they identify a preferred manner of address.

Communicate back to your patients with whatever medium they use to communicate with you. Call back if your patient calls. Answer e-mails in letter style rather than in acronyms and abbreviations. Older patients may be choosing their preferred mode of communication on the basis of personal preference, or they may be discreetly compensating for physical disabilities (e.g., using a phone because they have trouble reading computer screens because of declining visual ability).

Be aware of the strength of your therapeutic alliance at all times. When you are meeting the patient for the first time, you may want to engage another practitioner whom the patient trusts to reinforce and implement recommendations.

Look directly at the patient while you hear her history. Take notes with pen and paper or use an electronic devise that allows for eye contact.

Build personal connections by asking open-ended questions such as "Tell me, what brought you here?" Storytelling allows a patient to synthesize her life events and, eventually, to integrate her thoughts and emotions together.

Acknowledge when you do not know the answer to a question and then explain how you are going to handle the lack of certainty (e.g., "Scientists are currently studying this question"; "I will look up the answer"; "I will refer you for a consultation").

Provide recommendations in written and oral formats. Use clear and precise directions. Whenever possible, link an instruction to a regular daily routine. For example, direct the patient to "take sertraline one tablet (50 mg) after you eat breakfast" rather than "take sertraline 50 mg each day. Make sure you take it with food" (National Institute on Aging 2016).

ALLIANCE BUILDING WITH THE CAREGIVER OF AN OLDER ADULT

Consider Pat: She presented with Kate but only later divulged the complications of their relationship. Kate is Pat's identified caregiver, so you help Pat by building a therapeutic alliance with Kate. Imagine that Pat gives you permission to speak privately with Kate, who acknowledges that she cries at least a few times a week as she begs Pat to get out of bed. Although Pat can shower and dress herself, Kate has to ask multiple times before Pat will finally agree. Kate says, "I don't know what to do! She is just being mean at this point, and I fear it will only get worse. I fear that the rest of my life will be spent arguing with my mother." After you listen to Kate's fears and explain how depression is affecting Pat's behavior, Kate agrees to attend a local caregiver support group to learn more about how to take care of her mother.

The therapeutic alliance is also the key to building collaborative relationships between practitioners and caregivers; the well-being of the patient usually correlates with the well-being of her caregiver. We always offer caregivers our support and recognize their dedication. We remember that by the time they seek help, many are already nearly burned out. Preventing or alleviating caregiver burnout is a critical job for practitioners.

The first task is for practitioners to make sure they correctly understand the treatment goals of both caregiver and patient. Then, as roadblocks arise, they can explain how their recommendations will help achieve the caregiver's goals. Practitioners should also praise a caregiver for her dedication and hard work so she does not worry that accepting help would mean she is deficient or uncaring.

> In Pat's case, the real goal becomes not only to allay Kate's fears but also to engage her in Pat's treatment. When you speak to Kate again, she tells you, "Mom used to belong to a running club until Oscar died. Now she won't leave the house except when she comes with me to get the mail." You suggest, "So let's start with her trying to stay out longer when she gets the mail. Just ask her to take a walk in the backyard since she is already outside." Kate disagrees, "Mom will probably just say that's stupid." You respond, "I agree with you that she may turn down the idea. But you should at least try. If she says no, then we can figure out something else. We have nothing to lose by suggesting this."

Kate's concerns are similar to those of many caregivers we have seen. This case example demonstrates two important concepts: collaborative brainstorming and leeway. *Collaborative brainstorming* allows caregivers to share invaluable information about the patient, such as hobbies, interests, and her life story. Practitioners can then add this to their professional knowledge to help find effective, individualized treatment approaches. *Leeway* allows both providers and caregivers to try out new ideas in a safe environment. Implementing psychosocial interventions can be a trial-and-error process, as you tailor general guidelines to fit individual patients. Leeway is also helpful when caregivers appear to be "help rejecting." Structuring your recommendations with leeway built in can help them try new suggestions. Using collaborative brainstorming and leeway with caregivers can build a sense of mutual respect.

When caregivers do not implement your recommendations, you should consider that they may have burnout, but telling them they may have burnout can be tricky. We usually first suggest that they join a support group or seek individual counseling. Internet-based tools such as Link2Care (http://lists.caregiver.org/mailman/listinfo/link2care_discussion_lists.caregiver.org) and the Comprehensive Health Enhancement Support System (www.chess.wisc.edu/chess/home/home.aspx) can help caregivers who are unable to leave the home because of their duties (Collins and Swartz 2011). We also encourage caregivers to bring in someone else who can provide respite and become part of a patient's support network. One way to bring in another caregiver is to identify a backup proxy in case the primary caregiver is not available and then make sure the proxy is included in treatment planning.

QUICK TIPS FOR BUILDING A THERAPEUTIC ALLIANCE WITH CAREGIVERS

Use "we" and "us" to build a sense of unity between yourself and the caregiver: "We will figure out how to address your father's episodes of agitation."

Whenever possible, give caregivers time to think about your recommendations and encourage them to call you with any questions or concerns: "We have covered a lot of ground today, but we do not need to reach a decision. We can walk through this together."

Appreciate that caregivers often have high rates of medical illness and mental disorders, especially when caregivers are age 85 or older (Blazer 2000; Lee et al. 2008). Make sure a caregiver has a strong support network of her own, or caregiving itself can become a psychologically distressing experience: "We all need help when we are helping people."

Ensure the well-being of the caregiver. The better a caregiver does, the better a patient does: "When you return, I will ask about your health as a caregiver."

2

Addressing Behavioral and Mental Health Problems in Community Settings

Screening and Early Detection

Roberto is a 78-year-old man who emigrated from a small town in Mexico 4 years ago to live with his children. Two months ago he noticed blood in his urine; an urgent care center referred him to a urologist, who diagnosed Roberto with prostate cancer. A month ago, he underwent surgical removal of his prostate. Postoperatively, the urologist referred him to you for primary care.

Roberto arrives today, with his daughter, for his first primary care visit. Because both speak Spanish as their primary language, you ask for the assistance of an interpreter. While you await the arrival of the interpreter, Roberto takes the Spanish versions of the Patient Health Questionnaire 9-item depression scale (PHQ-9) and the Generalized Anxiety Disorder 7-Item Scale (GAD-7). His PHQ-9 total score is 4, but he has marked 2 (more than half the days) for the ninth item, "Thoughts that you would be better off dead or hurting yourself in some way." His GAD-7 total score is 7, suggesting mild anxiety.

In mental health care, a *screen* is an initial testing instrument used either to identify a previously undiagnosed disorder or to measure the severity of symptoms of a previously diagnosed disorder. There are three steps to using a screen: administering, scoring, and interpreting (Blais and Baer 2010). We discuss each of these concepts briefly here, with further details about how to correctly administer, score, and interpret several particular screens in Chapter 11, "Selected DSM-5 Assessment Measures." The instructions that accompany a mental health screen will usually explain if the screen is self-administered, caregiver administered, or practitioner administered. Scoring can be straightforward, such as when the practitioner adds up the numbers a patient has selected on the PHQ-9, or may require interpretation, such as when the practitioner determines whether the cube is drawn correctly on the Montreal Cognitive Assessment (MoCA).

An important part of mental health screening involves deciding which screens to use for which people. Something to keep in mind is that most screening instruments were validated with a particular group of people who may be quite different from the individual presenting to you. In today's clinical practice, it is common to encounter a person for whom, because of language, cultural heritage, cognitive ability, or other factors, the use of most screening instruments requires an act of translation. Translated screens can be valuable for an ethnically diverse population; however, if a screen has not been validated in a specific language, it should be used cautiously in the context of a clinical interview. Practitioners can always use screens in populations for which they have not been validated, but they should do so with humility and care, aware of the limits of the screening tool. In mental health settings, a thorough clinical interview or, in some cases, multiple interviews are needed to arrive at an accurate understanding of a person's mental distress.

Despite these caveats, we recommend screens both because they can save time in clinical interviews and because they allow you to communicate your findings to other practitioners. For example, if the result of a screening tool matches your findings from a brief interview and observation, both true positives and negatives, you can feel comfortable making a diagnosis based on the result. Then, when you record a diagnosis in your records, any consulting practitioners will have an objective sense of how you determined the diagnosis and its severity.

On the other hand, even well-validated screens like the PHQ-9 have limitations. Consider Roberto, who reported having frequent suicidal thoughts but responded mostly with 0 (not at all) or 1 (several days per week) to the other items on the PHQ-9. Roberto's responses are clues that you need to extend your inquiry.

When the interpreter arrives and you ask Roberto about his thoughts of being dead, he explains that in the past month he has become incontinent and impotent from surgery for prostate cancer but cannot afford to return to the urologist. He marked most of his answers on the PHQ-9 with a 0 or 1 because he assumed that most of his mood and somatic symptoms, such as fatigue and insomnia, were normal effects of surgery. After your brief interview, you are concerned that he may be minimizing his depressive symptoms, so you dedicate 15 minutes to exploring symptoms of depression and thoughts of suicide.

During your 15-minute mental health interview, Roberto explains that sometimes he feels so overwhelmed by the complications of his surgery that he stares at his pill bottles and thinks of overdosing on his medications. You diagnose him with major depressive disorder, start an antidepressant with low potential for lethality in overdose, and arrange for him to visit a depression care manager as part of your clinic's primary care mental health integration initiative. The depression care manager helps Roberto manage his depression and suicidal ideation. At your next visit, his PHQ-9 total score is 2, and he responds to the suicidal ideation question with 0. His GAD-7 total score has improved to 3.

Roberto's story has two major lessons. First, although his initial PHQ-9 score was a false negative, he benefited from screening, careful interpretation of the screen, and a follow-up interview. Looking at the individual items on the screen that are high yield (e.g., the suicidality item), in addition to the overall score, can help in both detecting false negatives and making a correct diagnosis. Second, Roberto's story illustrates how screening for mental health problems in primary care enables initiation of treatment before symptoms become severe. Early detection and treatment may prevent an adverse outcome, such as a suicide attempt due to an untreated severe major depressive episode or a driving accident due to undiagnosed neurocognitive disorder.

QUICK TIPS FOR SCREENING

Carefully follow the administration instructions for every screen, whether it is self-administered by the patient or administered by a caregiver or a practitioner.

Know the limitations of the screen, particularly regarding its validity for your patient population and the setting in which you work.

When a screen is consistent with a brief clinical interview, a mental health diagnosis can be made on the basis of its score.

If the screen, whether positive or negative, is inconsistent with a brief clinical interview or observation, a more detailed interview with the patient or an informant is necessary.

Assessment Tools for Use in a Brief Interview

To help a practitioner maximize his efficiency and effectiveness, Section III of DSM-5 (American Psychiatric Association 2013) includes assessment tools that a patient can fill out before a visit. The first form, the DSM-5 Self-Rated Level 1 Cross-Cutting Symptom Measure—Adult, is a psychiatric review of systems that correlates with DSM-5 criteria. For each major domain of mental illness, DSM-5 includes Level 2 Cross-Cutting Symptom Measures for a practitioner to administer. These tools can save time by allowing interviewers to structure their evaluations around the symptoms that concern a patient.

Diagnosis in Stages

In Chapter 9, we describe a stepwise approach to differential diagnosis from scratch. In this section, we describe how to clarify a diagnosis that you have identified using screening tools.

STAGE 1: CHARACTERIZATION OF A BEHAVIORAL OR MENTAL HEALTH PROBLEM IDENTIFIED BY A SCREENING TOOL

Vera is a 65-year-old woman with coronary artery disease and type 2 diabetes whom you have followed for the past 6 years in your clinic. At the end of her last visit, she reported feeling depressed about arguments with her children over money. You schedule an appointment for the following week to evaluate her depressive symptoms in detail. When she arrives for the visit, she completes the DSM-5 Self-Rated Level 1 Cross-Cutting Symptom Measure—Adult. She responds positively to questions about depressive and anxiety symptoms but negatively to the other questions, so you decide to focus your evaluation on determining whether Vera is experiencing a depressive or anxiety disorder and to administer the Level 2 tools for depression and anxiety.

As a practitioner reads through a patient's responses to assessment questions, he should consider which broad categories—such as mood, anxiety, substance use, personality, and cognition—fit the symptoms experienced by a patient. It is common to hear a chief complaint such as "I'm feeling sad," unconsciously decide that the most likely diagnosis is major depressive disorder, and immediately walk a patient through the DSM-5 criteria for major depressive disorder. Instead, you should listen to the patient's story, determine whether he spontaneously mentions the symptoms, and then explore further, asking the necessary questions to arrive at the specific diagnosis. A brief psychiatric review of systems should be performed to ensure that other symptoms or diagnoses have not been missed. Even experienced practitioners have been surprised to discover, after further investigation, that a seemingly depressed patient is actually having a mixed episode with manic and depressed features; or a depressed patient also has psychotic symptoms; or a person's depressed mood is caused by a medication, a substance of abuse, or another medical condition; or even that a depressed mood is a variant of normal behavior. Not every sad day is a depressed day.

After practitioners choose the potential diagnostic categories, they should differentiate among the mental disorders within those categories. For example, if a depressive disorder is the potential diagnosis, all the likely possibilities in that category, such as major depressive disorder, dysthymic disorder, and bipolar disorder, should be considered. This should be done systematically for each category, as modeled in Chapter 5, "The 15-Minute Older Adult Diagnostic Interview," and Chapter 6, "The 30-Minute Older Adult Diagnostic Interview."

STAGE 2: CONFIRMING A DIAGNOSIS USING DSM-5 CRITERIA

After using your assessment tools, you interview Vera. She shares with you that when she lived in East Berlin in the 1970s, she and her husband were wrongfully imprisoned for being spies. They were tortured, and Vera was raped in prison. When she reflected on those events over the years, she would experience intermittent sadness and anxiety. When her husband died 6 months ago, the sadness and anxiety became more frequent. At the end of your interview, your differential diagnosis, from most likely to least likely, includes major depressive disorder, generalized anxiety disorder, posttraumatic stress disorder (PTSD), and adjustment disorder with mixed anxiety and depressed mood.

After an initial evaluation, a practitioner should consider a broad differential diagnosis, include and exclude possibilities on the basis of the available information, and then confirm and treat the most likely diagnosis. One major difference between medical and psychiatric diagnostic approaches is that the diagnostic workup for a psychiatric disorder depends primarily on the clinical interview. Although laboratory work and neuroimaging can confirm a suspected diagnosis, the diagnosis must have first been considered on a thorough differential diagnosis.

When you interview Vera on the next visit, she reports that she has been drinking a shot of vodka at night for the past few years to help her sleep, but since her husband's death, she sometimes has 2–3 shots a couple of times per week to help her cope with her anxious thoughts, which range from worrying about her children to sometimes having nightmares about her rape. Suspecting PTSD, you administer the PTSD Checklist for DSM-5 (PCL-5), on which her score is 50. On the basis of the new information from Vera and her PCL-5 score, you eliminate adjustment disorder as a potential diagnosis, consider PTSD as more likely, and revisit the possibility of alcohol use disorder.

Over the next few months, Vera shares more of the suffering she experienced while living in East Berlin, her rape by a prison guard while the other guards laughed and humiliated her, and her immense relief when she was able to eventually escape and immigrate. You diagnose PTSD with comorbid major depressive disorder and alcohol use disorder, increase her antidepressant to the maximally tolerated dose, and refer her to a psychologist specializing in trauma disorders. Vera is able to entirely stop her alcohol use, and her PCL-5 score decreases to 30.

Confirming a diagnosis using DSM-5 criteria is often a trial-and-error process. Psychiatric diagnoses are based on longitudinal data, and your differential diagnosis will evolve as you get to know your patient better. Even from the start, remember that with DSM-5, you are not seeking a single diagnosis but rather developing a case formulation. In DSM-5, a case formulation "must involve a careful clinical history and concise summary of the social, psychological, and biological factors that may have contributed to developing a given mental disorder" and is never simply a checklist of symptoms (American Psychiatric Association 2013, p. 19). Instead, you have to include the "predisposing, precipitating, perpetuating, and protective factors" of a condition along with an "individual's cultural and social context" as you develop a comprehensive clinical case formulation (American Psychiatric Association 2013, p. 19). Psychiatric diagnosis teaches you humility and patience, as first impressions are often incorrect and best impressions develop along with the therapeutic relationship. Because it is not possible to cover all DSM-5 diagnoses in a brief visit, we focus on confirming or eliminating the most common diagnoses in older adults. Patients who do not respond well to initial treatment may require additional questioning about other DSM-5 diagnoses. For example, if a patient does not respond to multiple antidepressant trials, we consider other diagnostic possibilities, such as substance abuse or anxiety.

One useful technique in developing a differential diagnosis is to think about the clustering of mental health disorders, a frequent occurrence in many patients. Just as hypertension, hypercholesterolemia, diabetes, and obesity cluster in patients with metabolic syndrome, certain mental health disorders are frequently comorbid with other mental health disorders. For example, about 80% of respondents with PTSD in the National Comorbidity Survey had at least one other psychiatric disorder (Kessler et al. 1995), and 40% of participants in the National Epidemiologic Survey on Alcohol and Related Conditions with any drug use disorder had a comorbid mood disorder (Conway et al. 2006). The more mental health symptoms a patient has, the more likely it is that a cluster of mental health disorders, rather than a single disorder, will best explain his symptoms. Clusters can, unfortunately, mask redundant diagnoses. To discourage redundancy, many DSM-5 diagnoses are in a hierarchical relationship with each other. For example, in Vera's story, adjustment disorder was eliminated as a diagnostic possibility after recognizing that major depressive disorder and PTSD best explained her depressive and anxiety symptoms.

STAGE 3: EXPANSION OF THE DIFFERENTIAL DIAGNOSIS TO INCLUDE MEDICAL AND NEUROLOGICAL PROBLEMS

After doing well for 6 months on a regimen of trauma-focused psychotherapy and an antidepressant, Vera develops a resting tremor and bradykinesia. A movement disorders neurologist confirms the diagnosis of Parkinson's disease. During a follow-up visit in your clinic, Vera complains of some trouble balancing her checkbook. Because you know that cognitive impairment can occur even in the early stages of Parkinson's disease, you administer the MoCA with Vera because it is more sensitive than the Mini-Mental State Examination (MMSE) for impairment of executive functioning. Vera scores 20/30 and misses items related to executive functioning such as the Trails B and copying a cube. You suspect that she has mild neurocognitive disorder secondary to Parkinson's disease. Given her complicated psychiatric history, however, you also decide to refer her to a geriatric neuropsychologist for evaluation to confirm your diagnosis.

Clustering of mental health disorders with medical and neurological problems is quite common in older adults. Medical and neurological disorders such as thyroid disease, chronic obstructive pulmonary disease (COPD), Parkinson's disease, and Alzheimer's disease are frequently comorbid with psychiatric disorders. When older patients experience mental health symptoms for the first time, neurological disorders may be part of the differential diagnosis. For example, depression may be a prodrome for neurological disorders such as Parkinson's disease and Huntington's disease. Practitioners should be especially vigilant when patients exhibit neurological symptoms or report a family history of neurological disorders (Epping et al. 2016; Gustafsson et al. 2015; Vaccarino et al. 2011). Many medical and neurological disorders can be risk factors for mild neurocognitive disorder; when clinically indicated, a cognitive screen can identify a previously undiagnosed neurocognitive disorder.

By the time Vera is age 66, her medical history includes Parkinson's disease, COPD, coronary artery disease, hypertension, diabetes type 2, and obesity. Her score on the GAD-7 during her follow-up visit is 19. On further interview, she complains that she has discrete episodes of intermittent palpitations, shortness of breath, and an imminent sense of death in the context of trying to leave a crowded mall. She has significantly decreased her social outings because of this fear of "being trapped" in a public place. You diagnose panic disorder and agoraphobia. Vera does not want to take additional medication but is willing to resume treatment with a psychologist in the form of cognitive-behavioral therapy (CBT) for panic disorder.

When a patient complains of symptoms that can be attributed to a medical, neurological, or mental health disorder, the practitioner must consider the possibility that the symptoms may be due to any combination of these three categories, rather than one alone. For example, an older patient with COPD could have shortness of breath due to incomplete treatment of that disease with, or without, panic disorder. Sometimes frustration among multiple practitioners can arise, such as when a medical practitioner attributes shortness of breath to panic disorder, but the mental health practitioner attributes it to COPD. Practitioners need to recognize that both conditions may be triggering a patient's attacks of shortness of breath, in which case the patient's symptoms will not resolve until both the medical and mental disorders are treated.

Despite your best attempts to treat Vera's symptoms, she goes to the emergency department multiple times for her worsening panic attacks; at each visit, the emergency department doctors give her lorazepam and send her home. Two weeks later, she is found on the floor at home, having had a stroke, and is rushed to a local hospital, where she is discovered to have atrial fibrillation. You realize that what you believed to be panic attacks were episodes of atrial fibrillation, a common irregular heart rhythm that causes episodes of increased heart rate and breathlessness and can cause stroke.

A practitioner commits a common diagnostic error by assuming that a problem must be "psychiatric" because a patient behaves oddly or has a previous psychiatric history. If a practitioner assumes, for example, that a problem is "all in the patient's head" and neglects a thorough medical workup, a patient who appears anxious may not be assessed for pulmonary emboli, blood clots in the lung that can induce anxiety. Pulmonary emboli can be fatal; they are only one of the serious medical conditions that are neglected when a practitioner does not include medical and neurological disorders on the differential diagnosis. Practitioners should always perform a focused physical and neurological examination based on the patient's complaints and differential diagnosis.

> When Vera arrives for her first post-hospitalization visit, she ambulates with a walker. You perform a brief gait assessment and observe that she can tandem walk (i.e., pretend to walk on a tightrope) only three steps. She has a mild resting tremor. You become concerned about her ability to perform instrumental activities of daily living (IADLs) and activities of daily living (ADLs). Her daughter Gertrude confirms that Vera is struggling with IADLs because of slowed thinking and ADLs because of her new tremor. You also add to Vera's diagnoses mild neurocognitive disorder secondary to stroke and Parkinson's disease.

An important goal in the physical and neurological evaluation of older adults is the rapid assessment of functional status. For this age group, one of the most informative parts of the physical examination is the gait examination. This includes observation of a patient's gait speed, ability to walk on heels and tiptoes, and tandem walking. Practitioners can sense a patient's ability to function in the community on the basis of the gait assessment. For example, a practitioner can determine how easily a patient can walk, noticing shortness of breath or chest pain even if chronic, and any other symptoms that limit the patient's ability to get out in the community. It is also important to note whether the patient uses any assistive devices and, if so, whether this limits his ability to go out because the device may be difficult to transport or cause embarrassment. Assessment of ambulatory status is a useful tool that can quickly inform the practitioner about a patient's level of functioning and potential ability to participate in community activities.

The neurological examination can also provide invaluable information. The interpretation of this examination can be challenging for the nonspecialist; the key is to look for asymmetry and possible effects of any deficits on quality of life and/or functioning. The gait examination described earlier provides important information about the patient's ability to ambulate. An upper extremity examination can help clarify the patient's ability to perform various ADLs and socialization. An otherwise healthy older adult may struggle with some activities because of severe shoulder pain or experience social embarrassment due to worsening tremor. Tests for the upper extremities include palpation and observation for tremor and the assessment of rapid alternating movements, fine motor movements, coordination, range of motion (especially any limitations due to pain), and muscular strength. Common causes of tremor, a frequent complaint of many older people, include Parkinson's disease, parkinsonism, and essential tremor. One quick test to distinguish among these types of tremors is to examine the handwriting when patients are doing the written portions of cognitive screens such as the MoCA or the MMSE. Patients with essential tremor have large, shaky handwriting, whereas patients with Parkinson's disease or parkinsonism have smaller than normal writing and struggle to use the entire space despite encouragement to do so (Kaufman and Milstein 2013).

Treatment Planning and Care Coordination

When you discuss your diagnoses with Vera and her daughter, Gertrude expresses concern that Vera has been depressed since her stroke and does not want to leave home because she is embarrassed to use the walker and fears falling. After a diagnostic interview, you diagnose an episode of major depressive disorder and augment with a second antidepressant, mirtazapine. To improve Vera's functioning and address her negative feelings about using an assistive device, you suggest that she continue to work with her psychologist on CBT techniques that address her fear of falling. You also decide to refer Vera to physical therapy to reduce the risk of falls, a movement disorders neurologist to see whether her Parkinson's disease may improve from further treatment, and home health services.

Like the differential diagnosis, treatment planning is an evolving process that can be approached in several ways. The two most common approaches are the disease/disorder-based model and the symptom-based model. In the first, relevant diseases and disorders are listed with their appropriate treatments. The advantages of this model are that committing to a differential diagnosis can help practitioners think about treatments targeted to specific disorders, and they may find it more straightforward to include medical or neurological problems. The disadvantage is that symptoms that do not fit within the differential diagnosis may be excluded rather than explained.

In the symptom-based model, the practitioner first lists the various symptoms and then determines the differential diagnosis and appropriate treatment for each symptom. The advantage of this model is that organizing by symptoms allows comprehensive coverage of a patient's issues. The disadvantage is that the practitioner may not organize his thoughts sufficiently to come up with a diagnosis and therefore may not ask critical questions to confirm the diagnosis and determine the correct treatment. For example, a practitioner may fail to recognize a depressed episode as part of a related but undiagnosed condition, such as bipolar disorder or a depressive disorder secondary to hypothyroidism. The pitfall of the symptom-based approach is that it encourages practitioners to equate symptoms of mental illness to psychiatric disorders.

After the practitioner decides on a treatment plan, he should briefly communicate the diagnosis and its expected benefits and risks to the patient. Then the plan needs to be coordinated with the caregiver, the case manager, the staff at a setting such as a long-term-care facility, the referring practitioner, the primary care practitioner, and any others who are already involved or who need to become involved.

Opportunities to Integrate Behavioral Health Care

Integrating primary care and mental health has always been important, but recent research has confirmed the value. One analysis found that every $1.00 spent on primary care mental health integration saves about $6.50 in health care costs (Unützer et al. 2013). Examples of mental health integration in primary care include the Improving Mood–Promoting Access to Collaborative Treatment (IMPACT) and Prevention of Suicide in Primary Care Elderly: Collaborative Trial (PROSPECT) models. Both models rely on a physician extender, such as a care manager or a health specialist, specifically trained to deliver interventions for depression within the primary care setting. Studies of the IMPACT and PROSPECT models find that depression and suicidal ideation rates in older adults are reduced when mental health services are integrated into primary care (Bruce et al. 2004; Unützer et al. 2006).

Innovative models are also starting to integrate physical and mental health care in community-based settings. In the patient-centered primary care medical home, primary and

subspecialty care are based in the patient's own home to provide readily accessible, coordinated services. A key compo-
nent of the medical home is the psychiatric consultation
(Unützer et al. 2013). The Healthy Aging Brain Medical
Home is one such model that focuses on the comprehensive
care of mental health disorders in older adults; preliminary
evidence indicates that when behavioral health and primary
care are integrated, depression and dementia in older adults
can improve (LaMantia et al. 2015). The Care Partners project
is studying how to treat depression in older adults in community-based settings such as caregiver support groups,
adult day health, and churches (AIMS Center 2016). Delivering mental health services to medical homes and community-
based settings may be the future of mental health treatment
in older adults.

CHAPTER 3

The Diagnostic Ds

*The Building Blocks for Diagnosing
Mental Health Disorders
in Older Adults*

EXPLAINING an older person's mental distress as a single mental disorder is often challenging. Of course, simple is better; it is ideal to unify every symptom under a single diagnosis. However, a single diagnosis can be too simplistic; if you do not diagnose each medical and mental disorder a person is experiencing, you may misunderstand the nature of her distress, and your subsequent treatment will miss the mark. For example, if you neglect a patient's narcissistic character traits or her food insecurity, treating her depressive episode will prove challenging.

The key to diagnosing a patient with a complex presentation is to be open to possibilities. Start with the common disorders while keeping others in mind. In this chapter, we demonstrate, using three case examples, how you can focus on various clinical presentations of the diagnostic Ds—the six common disorders among older adults—while remembering alternative diagnoses. Understanding these six common disorders is critical because they represent the majority of mental health diagnoses in older adults.

For all DSM-5 criteria sets, ICD-9-CM and ICD-10-CM notes have been omitted for ease of reference. Please see DSM-5 for the complete criteria sets and accompanying text, including any recording procedures and coding notes.

THE SIX DIAGNOSTIC Ds

Delirium—an acute disturbance in attention and cognition

Drugs—prescribed medications, over-the-counter medications, illicit substances, alcohol, herbal medications, or supplements that may cause or exacerbate mental disorders

Diseases of medical or neurological origin—conditions that may explain or exacerbate mental disorders

Disrupted sleep—disturbances of the ability to initiate and maintain sleep and wakefulness

Depressive disorders—disturbances of mood

Dementia and other neurocognitive disorders—progressive cognitive deficits that degrade a person's independence

We typically start by considering delirium because it is both the most inclusive and the most reversible disorder. We work down the list step by step to the final D, dementia and other major neurocognitive disorders, the least reversible disorders. Along the way, we try to avoid these common errors:

- Diagnosing an irreversible disorder, such as Alzheimer's disease, when a patient actually has a potentially reversible condition, such as mild neurocognitive disorder due to benzodiazepine use
- Failure to diagnose a new-onset medical or neurological disorder that is comorbid with psychiatric disorders, such as when a patient has previously undiagnosed Parkinson's disease and presents with cognitive impairment and depression
- Making multiple diagnoses when a single one better explains all symptoms, such as when a hospitalized patient exhibiting sudden-onset mood, cognitive, and psychotic problems is diagnosed with Alzheimer's disease and major depressive disorder with psychotic features instead of with delirium

Delirium

Three years ago, Anni, a 75-year-old woman, was diagnosed with mild memory problems. Two weeks ago, she was hospitalized with pneumonia. She became confused and agitated, and although she was calmed by high doses of lorazepam and olanzapine, she rarely knew the year and could not recognize her husband, Matias. He brings her to your clinic for a post-hospitalization visit. He is concerned that Anni remains confused and wonders whether she developed dementia while hospitalized.

During your interview, you observe that Anni seems slightly drowsy but is awake throughout. She is oriented to herself and her husband but thinks the year is 1952 and she is back in her childhood home. Anni is not able to complete the tapping A task from the Montreal Cognitive Assessment (MoCA) successfully, stopping halfway through because she forgot what the task was. You administer a Short Confusion Assessment Method (Short CAM), a brief diagnostic test for delirium. The Short CAM confirms your concern that Anni is still lethargic and has delirium. Your repeat medical workup for an infection is negative. You reassure Matias that Anni has delirium that needs to resolve and provide him with tips to manage Anni's delirium at home. You teach Matias that until Anni's delirium resolves, you cannot comment on whether Anni has dementia.

When a patient presents with cognitive impairment, we first evaluate for delirium (Box 3–1), a reversible cause of cognitive impairment and a medical emergency that carries a high risk of mortality if left untreated. Delirium can take days to months to completely resolve. Older adults, especially those who had mild or major neurocognitive disorder prior to the episode of delirium, may not return to their baseline cognition and therefore will have a new cognitive baseline (Inouye 2006). The CAM is a brief questionnaire, available in 4-item and 10-item versions, that can be helpful for the detection of delirium (Inouye et al. 1990).

Box 3–1. Diagnostic Criteria for Delirium

A. A disturbance in attention (i.e., reduced ability to direct, focus, sustain, and shift attention) and awareness (reduced orientation to the environment).

B. The disturbance develops over a short period of time (usually hours to a few days), represents a change from baseline attention and awareness, and tends to fluctuate in severity during the course of a day.

C. An additional disturbance in cognition (e.g., memory deficit, disorientation, language, visuospatial ability, or perception).

D. The disturbances in Criteria A and C are not better explained by another preexisting, established, or evolving neurocognitive disorder and do not occur in the context of a severely reduced level of arousal, such as coma.

E. There is evidence from the history, physical examination, or laboratory findings that the disturbance is a direct physiological consequence of another medical condition, substance intoxication or withdrawal (i.e., due to a drug of abuse or to a medication), or exposure to a toxin, or is due to multiple etiologies.

Specify whether:

Substance intoxication delirium: This diagnosis should be made instead of substance intoxication when the symptoms in Criteria A and C predominate in the clinical picture and when they are sufficiently severe to warrant clinical attention.

Substance withdrawal delirium: This diagnosis should be made instead of substance withdrawal when the symptoms in Criteria A and C predominate in the clinical picture and when they are sufficiently severe to warrant clinical attention.

Medication-induced delirium: This diagnosis applies when the symptoms in Criteria A and C arise as a side effect of a medication taken as prescribed.

Delirium due to another medical condition: There is evidence from the history, physical examination, or laboratory findings that the disturbance is attributable to the physiological consequences of another medical condition.

Delirium due to multiple etiologies: There is evidence from the history, physical examination, or laboratory findings that the delirium has more than one etiology (e.g., more than one etiological medical condition; another medical condition plus substance intoxication or medication side effect).

Specify if:

Acute: Lasting a few hours or days.

Persistent: Lasting weeks or months.

Specify if:

Hyperactive: The individual has a hyperactive level of psychomotor activity that may be accompanied by mood lability, agitation, and/or refusal to cooperate with medical care.

Hypoactive: The individual has a hypoactive level of psychomotor activity that may be accompanied by sluggishness and lethargy that approaches stupor.

Mixed level of activity: The individual has a normal level of psychomotor activity even though attention and awareness are disturbed. Also includes individuals whose activity level rapidly fluctuates.

Drugs

You reassure Matias that Anni's delirium will likely improve. Indeed, 2 weeks later, Anni recognizes her husband and knows the year. She is frustrated, however, because poor concentration and lethargy prevent her from pursuing favorite hobbies such as reading and knitting. You review Anni's medication list, which includes the following prescriptions, some of which were prescribed by her previous primary care practitioner and the hospital physicians: cyclobenzaprine and tramadol for chronic pain, over-the-counter Tylenol PM and temazepam for sleep, clonazepam for anxiety, and diphenhydramine for seasonal allergies, plus olanzapine and as-needed lorazepam for agitation.

Concerned that the many different drugs Anni is taking may be contributing to her cognitive impairment, you initially stop the as-needed lorazepam because benzodiazepines are known to worsen delirium. Then you taper the olanzapine and switch her diphenhydramine to nasal saline and fluticasone sprays because both olanzapine and diphenhydramine are centrally acting. After repeated psychoeducation over three visits about how her pain medications, hypnotics, and benzodiazepines are contributing to her cognitive impairment, Anni agrees to pursue cognitive-behavioral therapy (CBT) for pain and anxiety in order to eventually stop cyclobenzaprine, tramadol, Tylenol PM, and benzodiazepines. She also agrees to stop drinking two glasses of wine every night. Three months after you first see her, Anni is taking only clonazepam and temazepam and reports that she is now able to knit some simple patterns again.

Drugs, whether prescribed medications, over-the-counter medications, alcohol, or illicit substances, are potentially reversible causes of cognitive impairment. Classes of prescribed medications that commonly contribute to cognitive impairment include pain medications (particularly opioids and those with anticholinergic properties), benzodiazepines, anticholinergics, antihistamines (including those sold over the counter), and sedative-hypnotics. Practitioners should also ask patients about use of alcohol, marijuana, illicit drugs, herbal medications, supplements, and over-the-counter medications, all of which can contribute to cognitive impairment. In Anni's case, multiple drugs are contributing to her cognitive impairment, so her DSM-5 diagnosis (American Psychiatric Association 2013) is mild neurocognitive disorder secondary to substance/medication use.

Diseases of Medical or Neurological Origin

> During your medical review of Anni's systems, she reports frequent tremors and inconsistent use of her continuous positive airway pressure (CPAP) machine. You are concerned about Parkinson's disease because her tremor has persisted despite stopping the olanzapine, and you refer her to a specialist in movement disorders for evaluation. He diagnoses essential tremor rather than Parkinson's disease and prescribes propranolol. You refer Anni to a primary care psychologist to improve her compliance with the CPAP. Over the next 2 months, Anni's CPAP compliance improves from 37% to 84%. She reports decreased lethargy and improved concentration, although she continues to take daytime naps for 1–2 hours each day and still struggles to use more complex knitting patterns.

Medical and neurological disorders other than delirium and major neurocognitive disorder are common causes of cognitive impairment. DSM-5 lists various causes of neurocognitive disorders, including those that affect the brain, such as stroke, traumatic brain injury, Parkinson's disease, and Huntington's disease. Other important conditions to investigate and manage are those that are potentially reversible, including obstructive sleep apnea (OSA), vitamin B_{12} deficiency, and hypothyroidism. Untreated sleep apnea can lead to attentional difficulties and daytime somnolence that cause significant underperformance on cognitive screening, which then can result in the misdiagnosis of dementia. In Anni's case, we first excluded Parkinson's disease, a potential neurological cause that might have explained her cognitive symptoms, and also looked for a medical problem (OSA) that explained or exacerbated her cognitive problems. Her DSM-5 diagnosis is mild neurocognitive disorder secondary to medical disorder.

Dementia and Other Neurocognitive Disorders

MILD NEUROCOGNITIVE DISORDER

> You successfully taper off Anni's temazepam, but as you begin tapering off her clonazepam, she complains of worsening anxiety and feeling "blue." She confesses concern that she is developing dementia because she continues to struggle with favorite activities and paying the bills. She says, "I

don't remember what I did more than 5 minutes ago." She remains housebound because of chronic pain. As you problem solve, Anni eventually agrees to a trial of venlafaxine to treat her depression, anxiety, and pain. She also attends booster CBT sessions for anxiety. After 2 months of combined treatment with an antidepressant and CBT, Anni returns "mostly to the way I was before I was in the hospital." On the Patient Health Questionnaire 9-item depression scale (PHQ-9), Anni's score is 2, which is consistent with the absence of depressive symptoms. She is able to pursue most activities without difficulty, although she notes intermittent difficulty with word finding and recalling details of recent events a few weeks later. Her MoCA score is 24/30. She loses points in the domains of attention, word fluency, and delayed recall; however, these stable deficits appear mild and do not affect her functioning significantly, as she is able to compensate by making checklists and programming reminders into her cell phone. Now that you have optimized her medication regimen and addressed the medical and mental health issues contributing to her cognitive impairment, you tentatively diagnose Anni with mild neurocognitive disorder and refer her for detailed neuropsychological evaluation to make sure she does not have dementia (major neurocognitive disorder). The geriatric neuropsychologist confirms your diagnosis because Anni performs 1–2 standard deviations below the mean in the domains of memory and executive functioning.

Depressive disorders, ranging from depressive episode with insufficient symptoms to major depressive disorder, are often accompanied by subjective cognitive complaints. In some cases, the cognitive deficits will resolve, but in others they will persist. The cognitive impairment can range from mild difficulty paying attention to an inability to complete complex activities or to a dementia-like picture historically referred to as pseudodementia. Practitioners should suspect depression as a significant cause of cognitive impairment when patients' cognitive complaints are significantly worse than their cognitive and functional performance on objective measures.

Depression should be aggressively treated both because it is an independent risk for dementia (Byers and Yaffe 2011) and because its presence can compromise an accurate diagnosis of a neurocognitive disorder. In Anni's case, her depressive symptoms were aggressively treated before she was referred for neuropsychological evaluation and diagnosed with mild neurocognitive disorder (Box 3–2) due to Alzheimer's disease. However, patients with atypical presentation and/or failure to respond to multiple trials of antidepressants should be referred for neuropsychological evaluation because behavioral symptoms can be the presenting feature of atypical major neurocognitive disorders such as those due to frontotemporal dementia (Lanata and Miller 2016).

Box 3–2.   Diagnostic Criteria for Mild Neurocognitive Disorder

---

A. Evidence of modest cognitive decline from a previous level of performance in one or more cognitive domains (complex attention, executive function, learning and memory, language, perceptual-motor, or social cognition) based on:

1. Concern of the individual, a knowledgeable informant, or the clinician that there has been a mild decline in cognitive function; and

2. A modest impairment in cognitive performance, preferably documented by standardized neuropsychological testing or, in its absence, another quantified clinical assessment.

B. The cognitive deficits do not interfere with capacity for independence in everyday activities (i.e., complex instrumental activities of daily living such as paying bills or managing medications are preserved, but greater effort, compensatory strategies, or accommodation may be required).

C. The cognitive deficits do not occur exclusively in the context of a delirium.

D. The cognitive deficits are not better explained by another mental disorder (e.g., major depressive disorder, schizophrenia).

Specify whether due to:
Alzheimer's disease ([DSM-5] pp. 611–614)
Frontotemporal lobar degeneration ([DSM-5] pp. 614–618)
Lewy body disease ([DSM-5] pp. 618–621)
Vascular disease ([DSM-5] pp. 621–624)
Traumatic brain injury ([DSM-5] pp. 624–627)
Substance/medication use ([DSM-5] pp. 627–632)
HIV infection ([DSM-5] pp. 632–634)
Prion disease ([DSM-5] pp. 634–636)
Parkinson's disease ([DSM-5] pp. 636–638)
Huntington's disease ([DSM-5] pp. 638–641)
Another medical condition ([DSM-5] pp. 641–642)
Multiple etiologies ([DSM-5] pp. 642–643)
Unspecified ([DSM-5] p. 643)

Specify:

Without behavioral disturbance: If the cognitive disturbance is not accompanied by any clinically significant behavioral disturbance.

With behavioral disturbance *(specify disturbance):* If the cognitive disturbance is accompanied by a clinically significant behavioral disturbance (e.g., psychotic symptoms, mood disturbance, agitation, apathy, or other behavioral symptoms).

MAJOR NEUROCOGNITIVE DISORDER (DEMENTIA)

Anni returns for her annual follow-up visit 3 years later. Matias reports concern about her inability to pay bills and to remember shared memories. Both he and Anni deny any mood symptoms, but she now has trouble with paperwork and recently got lost for a couple of hours when driving to a familiar area. You readminister the MoCA. She scores 20/30, a significant decline from her previous score of 24/30. She misses 4 out of 5 words on delayed recall and is unable to recall any words even with category or multiple-choice cueing. Her PHQ-9 score is 3. You repeat lab work for any potentially reversible cause of cognitive impairment, and the results are within normal limits. You diagnose major neurocognitive disorder and prescribe donepezil.

Anni was previously diagnosed with mild neurocognitive disorder because her cognitive decline did not lead to functional deficits and she was able to compensate. The latest development of *irreversible* functional decline secondary to her *irreversible* cognitive decline, however, points to a diagnosis of major neurocognitive disorder (Box 3–3). To make this diagnosis, a practitioner must determine that a patient's deficits represent a decline from the premorbid cognitive and functional baseline. One common reason a patient can be misdiagnosed with major neurocognitive disorder is that practitioners do not recognize that the patient has low educational attainment, an undiagnosed neurodevelopmental or chronic mental disorder, or baseline poor functional attainment. The other key to making an accurate diagnosis of major neurocognitive disorder is that functional decline must be the result of a cognitive decline. A common diagnostic error is to notice that a patient has worsening function without realizing that the impaired functioning is due to a medical condition such as arthritis rather than cognitive decline (Table 3–1). Deciding whether functional decline is due to physical causes and/or cognitive causes can be quite challenging in the oldest old, those who are at least age 85, because symptoms often coexist. One way practitioners can decide whether patients with physical disabilities also have a cognitive deficit is to ask a patient to describe, step by step, how she would perform a task such as cooking or going to the grocery store if she were physically capable.

Box 3–3. Diagnostic Criteria for Major Neurocognitive Disorder

A. Evidence of significant cognitive decline from a previous level of performance in one or more cognitive domains (complex attention, executive function, learning and memory, language, perceptual-motor, or social cognition) based on:

1. Concern of the individual, a knowledgeable informant, or the clinician that there has been a significant decline in cognitive function; and

2. A substantial impairment in cognitive performance, preferably documented by standardized neuropsychological testing or, in its absence, another quantified clinical assessment.

B. The cognitive deficits interfere with independence in everyday activities (i.e., at a minimum, requiring assistance with complex instrumental activities of daily living such as paying bills or managing medications).

C. The cognitive deficits do not occur exclusively in the context of a delirium.

D. The cognitive deficits are not better explained by another mental disorder (e.g., major depressive disorder, schizophrenia).

Specify whether due to:
Alzheimer's disease ([DSM-5] pp. 611–614)
Frontotemporal lobar degeneration ([DSM-5] pp. 614–618)
Lewy body disease ([DSM-5] pp. 618–621)
Vascular disease ([DSM-5] pp. 621–624)
Traumatic brain injury ([DSM-5] pp. 624–627)
Substance/medication use ([DSM-5] pp. 627–632)
HIV infection ([DSM-5] pp. 632–634)
Prion disease ([DSM-5] pp. 634–636)
Parkinson's disease ([DSM-5] pp. 636–638)
Huntington's disease ([DSM-5] pp. 638–641)
Another medical condition ([DSM-5] pp. 641–642)
Multiple etiologies ([DSM-5] pp. 642–643)
Unspecified ([DSM-5] p. 643)

Specify:

Without behavioral disturbance: If the cognitive disturbance is not accompanied by any clinically significant behavioral disturbance.

With behavioral disturbance *(specify disturbance):* If the cognitive disturbance is accompanied by a clinically significant behavioral disturbance (e.g., psychotic symptoms, mood disturbance, agitation, apathy, or other behavioral symptoms).

Specify current severity:

Mild: Difficulties with instrumental activities of daily living (e.g., housework, managing money).

Moderate: Difficulties with basic activities of daily living (e.g., feeding, dressing).

Severe: Fully dependent.

Depressive Disorders

BEREAVEMENT

> Jia is an 86-year-old woman with hypertension who reports sadness after her husband of 65 years passed away 2 weeks ago from a heart attack. She cries easily and often. She sometimes hears her husband's voice talking to her. Jia thinks daily about when she will die and join her husband, but she denies any intent to hurt herself. She is still able to enjoy the time she spends with her friends and family, although she cries when someone mentions her husband's name.

Bereavement or grief is the emotional, cognitive, and functional response experienced by a person following the death of a family member or friend. What constitutes normal bereavement or grief varies widely depending on cultural, social, and religious expectations. On the psychological assessment tool called the Holmes-Rahe Stress Scale, the death of a spouse is considered to be the most stressful event in a person's life, earning a score of 100 of a possible 100 points (Holmes and Rahe 1967). In DSM-IV-TR (American Psychiatric Association 2000), the criteria for major depressive disorder included a bereavement exclusion that allowed practitioners to wait up to 2 months after the death before making the diagnosis of major depressive disorder. The bereavement exclusion has been removed in DSM-5. The ensuing controversy indicates how difficult it can be to determine if a person's bereavement is a normal variant or a pathologi-

TABLE 3–1. Common diagnostic pitfalls for cognitive impairment

1. Failure to rapidly diagnose delirium because severe cognitive deficits are expected, even though they can be quite mild, such as when the patient has trouble completing a sentence but then finishes it a few seconds later or is slightly drowsy but able to answer questions coherently during the interview.

2. Assuming that delirium is not present because an infectious workup and head imaging are negative. Common causes of delirium that can yield a negative medical workup, such as environmental changes (being in the hospital), insomnia, untreated pain, or medications such as anesthesia, may be missed.

3. Failure to rapidly diagnose delirium in hospitalized patients with major neurocognitive disorder because of an assumption that new-onset behavioral disturbances are part of a premorbid psychiatric disorder.

4. Becoming distracted by the more prominent mood and/or psychotic symptoms of delirium or major neurocognitive disorder with behavioral disturbance without evaluating for cognitive changes.

5. Incorrectly diagnosing older patients with major neurocognitive disorder as a result of forgetting to evaluate for potentially reversible causes of cognitive impairment such as medical disorders, depression, and drugs.

cal state. In DSM-5, the distinction depends on whether the bereavement interferes with ordinary functioning. Making this decision correctly has therapeutic value because normal bereavement is time limited and resolves on its own, whereas individuals with persistent complex bereavement disorder, a proposed diagnostic entity in DSM-5, may benefit from further intervention, such as psychotherapy. Because Jia is still able to function at the same level as prior to her husband's death, she is probably experiencing normal bereavement.

MAJOR DEPRESSIVE DISORDER

Two weeks later, Jia comes with her son Chongan for a follow-up visit. Since the last visit, he has become concerned that Jia lies in bed most of the day, watching TV and knitting. Instead of eating solid foods, she is subsisting on liquid nutritional supplements and has lost 10 pounds. She told Chongan that she no longer cares about living. During your interview, Jia denies any intent to hurt herself, explaining that she switched to the nutritional supplements because she feared other food was poisoned. She denies hearing any voices, except occasionally her husband's voice comforting her. You prescribe an antidepressant. When you see her a month later, her mood symptoms are improved, but she continues to drink only nutritional supplements, so you prescribe an adjunctive antipsychotic. Two days after beginning to take the antipsychotic, Jia begins to eat solid food again.

DSM-5 defines major depressive disorder (Box 3–4) as one or more major depressive episodes in the absence of a hypomanic, mixed, or manic episode or mood-incongruent psychotic symptoms. Using DSM-IV-TR, practitioners could delay a diagnosis of major depressive disorder for 2 months in the setting of bereavement. DSM-5 removed this delay because subsequent research found no benefit in delaying the diagnosis of major depressive disorder in adults who were grieving. For a patient whose grief has become a full depressive episode, DSM-5 removed the 2-month bereavement delay so treatment can begin sooner. However, DSM-5 also makes clear that the practitioner still has to make a prudent judgment when determining if a person is grieving, depressed, or both (American Psychiatric Association 2015a). Even while making this determination, the practitioner should comfort a grieving patient.

Box 3–4. Diagnostic Criteria for Major Depressive Disorder

A. Five (or more) of the following symptoms have been present during the same 2-week period and represent a change from previous functioning; at least one of the symptoms is either (1) depressed mood or (2) loss of interest or pleasure.
Note: Do not include symptoms that are clearly attributable to another medical condition.

1. Depressed mood most of the day, nearly every day, as indicated by either subjective report (e.g., feels sad, empty, hopeless) or observation made by others (e.g., appears tearful). (**Note:** In children and adolescents, can be irritable mood.)

2. Markedly diminished interest or pleasure in all, or almost all, activities most of the day, nearly every day (as indicated by either subjective account or observation).

3. Significant weight loss when not dieting or weight gain (e.g., a change of more than 5% of body weight in a month), or decrease or increase in appetite nearly every day. (**Note:** In children, consider failure to make expected weight gain.)

4. Insomnia or hypersomnia nearly every day.

5. Psychomotor agitation or retardation nearly every day (observable by others, not merely subjective feelings of restlessness or being slowed down).

6. Fatigue or loss of energy nearly every day.

7. Feelings of worthlessness or excessive or inappropriate guilt (which may be delusional) nearly every day (not merely self-reproach or guilt about being sick).

8. Diminished ability to think or concentrate, or indecisiveness, nearly every day (either by subjective account or as observed by others).

9. Recurrent thoughts of death (not just fear of dying), recurrent suicidal ideation without a specific plan, or a suicide attempt or a specific plan for committing suicide.

B. The symptoms cause clinically significant distress or impairment in social, occupational, or other important areas of functioning.

C. The episode is not attributable to the physiological effects of a substance or another medical condition.

Note: Criteria A–C represent a major depressive episode.

Note: Responses to a significant loss (e.g., bereavement, financial ruin, losses from a natural disaster, a serious medical illness or disability) may include the feelings of intense sadness, rumination about the loss, insomnia, poor appetite, and weight loss noted in Criterion A, which may resemble a depressive episode. Although such symptoms may be understandable or considered appropriate to the loss, the presence of a major depressive episode in addition to the normal response to a significant loss should also be carefully considered. This decision inevitably requires the exercise of clinical judgment based on the individual's history and the cultural norms for the expression of distress in the context of loss.[1]

D. The occurrence of the major depressive episode is not better explained by schizoaffective disorder, schizophrenia, schizophreniform disorder, delusional disorder, or other specified and unspecified schizophrenia spectrum and other psychotic disorders.

E. There has never been a manic episode or a hypomanic episode.
   Note: This exclusion does not apply if all of the manic-like or hypomanic-like episodes are substance-induced or are attributable to the physiological effects of another medical condition.

In recording the name of a diagnosis, terms should be listed in the following order: major depressive disorder, single or recurrent episode, severity/psychotic/remission specifiers, followed by as many of the following specifiers without codes that apply to the current episode.

Specify:
   With anxious distress ([DSM-5] p. 184)
   With mixed features ([DSM-5] pp. 184–185)
   With melancholic features ([DSM-5] p. 185)
   With atypical features ([DSM-5] pp. 185–186)
   With mood-congruent psychotic features ([DSM-5] p. 186)
   With mood-incongruent psychotic features ([DSM-5] p. 186)
   With catatonia ([DSM-5] p. 186)
   With peripartum onset ([DSM-5] pp. 186–187)
   With seasonal pattern (recurrent episode only) ([DSM-5] pp. 187–188)

Regardless of whether or not older individuals are explicitly grieving, depressive disorder can be more difficult to diagnose in older adults than in younger adults. Most older adults have experienced losses of various kinds. Instead of appearing sad, some older patients may manifest depression by being somatically preoccupied and withdrawn, whereas others may present with irritability and poor sleep, which

----

[1]In distinguishing grief from a major depressive episode (MDE), it is useful to consider that in grief the predominant affect is feelings of emptiness and loss, while in an MDE it is persistent depressed mood and the inability to anticipate happiness or pleasure. The dysphoria in grief is likely to decrease in intensity over days to weeks and occurs in waves, the so-called pangs of grief. These waves tend to be associated with thoughts or reminders of the deceased. The depressed mood of an MDE is more persistent and not tied to specific thoughts or preoccupations. The pain of grief may be accompanied by positive emotions and humor that are uncharacteristic of the pervasive unhappiness and misery characteristic of an MDE. The thought content associated with grief generally features a preoccupation with thoughts and memories of the deceased, rather than the self-critical or pessimistic ruminations seen in an MDE. In grief, self-esteem is generally preserved, whereas in an MDE feelings of worthlessness and self-loathing are common. If self-derogatory ideation is present in grief, it typically involves perceived failings vis-à-vis the deceased (e.g., not visiting frequently enough, not telling the deceased how much he or she was loved). If a bereaved individual thinks about death and dying, such thoughts are generally focused on the deceased and possibly about "joining" the deceased, whereas in an MDE such thoughts are focused on ending one's own life because of feeling worthless, undeserving of life, or unable to cope with the pain of depression.

may lead to mistaken diagnoses of somatic and bipolar disorders, respectively. Typically, patients with somatic disorders are fearful or preoccupied about being ill and make frequent use of medical care without being reassured. Patients who have never had a diagnosis of bipolar disorder or have never taken psychotropic medications to treat bipolar disorder are unlikely to experience initial onset after age 60.

Older adults experiencing depression, however, are more likely than younger adults to have psychotic features, such as auditory or visual hallucinations, delusions, and paranoia. It is important to distinguish psychosis from bereavement and expressions of mourning that are normal for the person's cultural background. Hearing the voice of a deceased family member or friend is not necessarily psychosis; depending on the person's cultural and religious background, these voices may be benign or even comforting. Benign voices are typically memories of the past or messages of consolation, such as "Someday we will be together in heaven." Voices that command or speak to the patient about derogatory material, especially if the patient and the deceased had a positive relationship, require further exploration for depressive symptoms. Because Jia is both depressed and paranoid enough that she has stopped eating solid food, she now meets the criteria for major depressive disorder with mood-congruent psychotic features.

MAJOR NEUROCOGNITIVE DISORDER WITH BEHAVIORAL DISTURBANCE: APATHY

> After 3 months of a therapeutic trial of an antidepressant, Jia returns to your office for a follow-up visit. Chongan expresses concern that his mother "just sits there," usually watching TV. Her score on the Geriatric Depression Scale (GDS) is 2/15. Her score on the MoCA is 20/30. On obtaining further history from Chongan, you learn that Jia's husband had taken over the bill paying and other complex activities prior to his death because Jia was "more stressed out." You diagnose her with major neurocognitive disorder due to possible Alzheimer's disease and determine that her withdrawn behavior is from apathy, a behavioral disturbance commonly seen in such cases.

Apathy is a common behavioral disturbance seen in various neurological and psychiatric disorders. Patients with apathy have difficulty pursuing activities because of amotivation and often appear disengaged even from emotionally meaningful discussions. These symptoms are due to deficits in the frontal lobes, an area of the brain that is important for motivation and planning of complex behavior. Apathy may occur in the absence of depression, or at least may not be completely explained by the severity of depressive symptoms observed. Neurological and psychiatric disorders associated with apathy include mild neurocognitive disorder, major neurocognitive disorder (dementia), stroke, Parkinson's disease, major depressive disorder, subsyndromal depression, and schizophrenia. The prevalence of apathy in Alzheimer's disease ranges from 36% to 88% (van Reekum et al. 2005). Caregivers can feel quite frustrated with patients who have apathy and are sitting like "a bump on a log" for hours. Sometimes, it can be clinically difficult to distinguish apathy from depression; patients may need to be empirically treated with an antidepressant to see whether their symptoms improve.

Disrupted Sleep

INSOMNIA

> Bill is a 72-year-old man you know well. At a routine visit, he requests a sleeping pill, saying that he has been having problems falling asleep for the past 2 years. Since he retired 3 months ago, his sleep problems have gotten progressively worse. He lies in bed for 3–4 hours before finally falling asleep around midnight. Then he wakes up a few times in the night and has trouble falling back to sleep. When you ask about his regular daytime activities, he says that he wakes up between 7 and 11 A.M., watches TV or uses the computer most of the day, and naps 1–2 hours every day.

Older adults, especially recently retired adults, frequently complain of insomnia because they lack stimulating daytime activities. After people stop working, they often lack an external structure for their daytime activities. Many spend hours in front of a TV or computer and frequently nap during the day. The combination of daytime napping and decreased exposure to natural light disrupts or degrades nighttime sleep. For older people with insomnia (Box 3–5), a practitioner should focus on both sleep hygiene (Table 3–2) and structuring daytime activities to ensure that retired adults remain mentally stimulated and socially active. A sleep diary can help a patient understand how much sleep she is actually getting. If you do not suspect a sleep disorder, it is reasonable to prescribe hypnotics for a short period of time—no more than a few months—while you work with the patient to implement sleep hygiene measures. About 40% of people with insomnia have a comorbid psychiatric disorder (Roth 2007), so practitioners should carefully evaluate comorbid depression and anxiety. CBT for insomnia (CBT-I) with a therapist or via the Internet can be quite helpful (Winkelman 2015).

Box 3–5. Diagnostic Criteria for Insomnia Disorder

A. A predominant complaint of dissatisfaction with sleep quantity or quality, associated with one (or more) of the following symptoms:

    1. Difficulty initiating sleep. (In children, this may manifest as difficulty initiating sleep without caregiver intervention.)

    2. Difficulty maintaining sleep, characterized by frequent awakenings or problems returning to sleep after awakenings. (In children, this may manifest as difficulty returning to sleep without caregiver intervention.)

    3. Early-morning awakening with inability to return to sleep.

B. The sleep disturbance causes clinically significant distress or impairment in social, occupational, educational, academic, behavioral, or other important areas of functioning.

C. The sleep difficulty occurs at least 3 nights per week.

D. The sleep difficulty is present for at least 3 months.

E. The sleep difficulty occurs despite adequate opportunity for sleep.

F. The insomnia is not better explained by and does not occur exclusively during the course of another sleep-wake disorder (e.g., narcolepsy, a breathing-related sleep disorder, a circadian rhythm sleep-wake disorder, a parasomnia).

G. The insomnia is not attributable to the physiological effects of a substance (e.g., a drug of abuse, a medication).

H. Coexisting mental disorders and medical conditions do not adequately explain the predominant complaint of insomnia.

Specify if:

    With non–sleep disorder mental comorbidity, including substance use disorders

    With other medical comorbidity

    With other sleep disorder

Specify if:

    Episodic: Symptoms last at least 1 month but less than 3 months.

    Persistent: Symptoms last 3 months or longer.

Recurrent: Two (or more) episodes within the space of 1 year.

Note: Acute and short-term insomnia (i.e., symptoms lasting less than 3 months but otherwise meeting all criteria with regard to frequency, intensity, distress, and/or impairment) should be coded as an other specified insomnia disorder.

TABLE 3–2.   Sleep hygiene guidelines

1. Establish regular bedtimes and wake-up times.

2. Go to bed only when sleepy.

3. Get out of bed after 20 minutes if you cannot sleep.

4. Avoid alcohol, caffeine, and nicotine for 4–6 hours before bedtime.

5. Use the bed only for sleep or sex.

6. Nap for no more than 30 minutes during the daytime.

7. Maintain a relaxing bedtime ritual.

8. Take a hot bath 1–2 hours before bedtime.

9. Avoid clock watching.

10. Exercise during the day.

11. Establish a comfortable space for sleep.

12. Stick to your regular routine even if you are tired.

BREATHING-RELATED SLEEP DISORDER

Bill implements your recommendations for sleep hygiene but also takes an over-the-counter melatonin supplement that his wife recommended. Despite these efforts, he continues to complain of daytime fatigue and notes, "My wife complains I snore." You wonder whether he may have OSA in addition to insomnia disorder. He scores 14 on the Epworth Sleepiness Scale (ESS), and his body mass index is 36. You refer him for polysomnography to confirm your suspicion of OSA.

Diagnosing OSA (Box 3–6) in older adults can be challenging, especially if they have a healthy habitus and do not snore. Typically, insomnia is one of the first signs of OSA in older adults. The ESS can be used to clarify the diagnosis of OSA; a positive score on this scale suggests the diagnosis, whereas a negative score makes the diagnosis of OSA less likely, albeit without entirely excluding the possibility of OSA. When you suspect that a patient has a breathing-related sleep disorder such as OSA, you should avoid or minimize the use of benzodiazepines or benzodiazepine derivatives, such as zolpidem, because these drugs may worsen apneic episodes.

Box 3–6.   Diagnostic Criteria for Obstructive Sleep Apnea Hypopnea

---

A. Either (1) or (2):

1. Evidence by polysomnography of at least five obstructive apneas or hypopneas per hour of sleep and either of the following sleep symptoms:

    a. Nocturnal breathing disturbances: snoring, snorting/gasping, or breathing pauses during sleep.

    b. Daytime sleepiness, fatigue, or unrefreshing sleep despite sufficient opportunities to sleep that is not better explained by another mental disorder (including a sleep disorder) and is not attributable to another medical condition.

2. Evidence by polysomnography of 15 or more obstructive apneas and/or hypopneas per hour of sleep regardless of accompanying symptoms.

Specify current severity:
   Mild: Apnea hypopnea index is less than 15.
   Moderate: Apnea hypopnea index is 15–30.
   Severe: Apnea hypopnea index is greater than 30.

On review of systems, Bill reports problems with feeling jittery, especially at night, and trouble lying still. On the basis of this additional information, you suspect Bill has restless legs syndrome (RLS) and decide to interview his wife. She complains that Bill started to kick her in his sleep about 2 years ago, and she now sleeps in a separate bed. You suspect that Bill also has periodic limb movement disorder (PLMD) and hope polysomnography will settle the diagnosis.

PERIODIC LIMB MOVEMENT DISORDER AND RESTLESS LEGS SYNDROME

PLMD and RLS are similar sleep disorders, and both can cause insomnia, so distinguishing between them is challenging. RLS is usually characterized by an urge to constantly move the legs when they are resting. PLMD is usually characterized by constant leg jerking or twitching after the patient is asleep. RLS can be diagnosed only on the basis of clinical history, whereas PLMD can be confirmed on polysomnography. Although about 80% of patients with RLS also have PLMD (National Institute of Neurological Disorders and Stroke 2015), patients with PLMD usually do not have RLS. The treatments for RLS and PLMD are quite similar. Table 3–3 compares the features of PLMD and RLS.

TABLE 3–3. Features of periodic limb movement disorder (PLMD) and restless legs syndrome (RLS)

	PLMD	RLS
Clinical features	Constant leg jerking or twitching Symptoms when patient is asleep Bed partner usually notices symptoms	Urge to constantly move the legs when they are resting and urge is worse at night Unpleasant sensations in legs Symptoms when patient is asleep Patient usually notices symptoms
Risk factors	Old age Renal disease Diabetes Peripheral neuropathy Pregnancy Iron deficiency anemia Family history Dopaminergic antagonists (certain types of antiemetics and antipsychotics) Antidepressants that increase serotonin	Old age Renal disease Diabetes Peripheral neuropathy Pregnancy Iron deficiency anemia Family history Dopaminergic antagonists (certain types of antiemetics and antipsychotics) Antidepressants that increase serotonin

TABLE 3–3. Features of periodic limb movement disorder (PLMD) and restless legs syndrome (RLS) *(continued)*

	PLMD	RLS
Diagnostic test	Clinical history Blood tests can help to identify potential causes but are not diagnostic Polysomnography	Clinical history Blood tests can help to identify potential causes but are not diagnostic
Treatment	Avoid caffeine Dopaminergic agonists Benzodiazepines and opiates (if not responsive to dopaminergic agents) Anticonvulsants	Dopaminergic agonists (first-line agents are pramipexole and ropinirole; avoid pergolide) Benzodiazepines and opiates (if not responsive to dopaminergic agents) Anticonvulsants (gabapentin enacarbil, pregabalin, carbamazepine)

Source. Aurora et al. 2012; National Institute of Neurological Disorders and Stroke 2015.

CHAPTER 4

Beyond the Diagnostic Ds

Other Common Clinical Challenges

Unusual Experiences, Irritability, and Labile Mood

The diagnostic Ds discussed in Chapter 3 provide a framework to diagnose and manage common mental health problems in older adults. In this chapter, we will cover the diagnostic workup and management of other common mental health problems in older adults. These common problems are mood changes such as irritability and labile mood, unusual experiences such as hallucinations and delusions, agitation and aggression, sexual dysfunction, and suicide and end-of-life concerns. These diagnoses should be included with the diagnostic Ds to ensure a comprehensive mental health assessment in the older adult.

DELIRIUM AND SUBSTANCE- AND MEDICATION-RELATED DISORDERS

While on service for the weekend, you are called to see Daniel, a 59-year-old man who was hospitalized a week ago for a chronic obstructive pulmonary disease (COPD) exacerbation and pneumonia. He has responded well to his antibiotic regimen, and his steroid taper was started 2 days ago. The nurses report that Daniel has not been sleeping well for the past 2 nights and has become increasingly agitated. His workup for delirium yesterday was negative. When you see Daniel, he is jumping up and down on the bed and announcing, "I am the son of God, and I will be the first man to fly!" You try to redirect Daniel, but he continues to talk rapidly about how he is in special communication with NASA to learn how to fly. He requires two intramuscular injections of haloperidol 0.5 mg to fall asleep. You call his daughter Samira, who tells you that when Daniel has required outpatient steroid tapers for his COPD in the past 2 years, he has occasionally "said some strange stuff, but it always goes away, so we just ignore him." Daniel requires low-dose oral haloperidol during the rest of his steroid taper; after that is completed, he returns to his baseline, so you stop the haloperidol.

The case example of Daniel illustrates the importance of recognizing medications as a potentially reversible cause of mania. Practitioners should always exclude delirium, medications, and illicit or over-the-counter substances as causes of sudden changes in behavior. In particular, when patients develop sudden-onset psychotic symptoms in an acute medical or surgical setting, delirium should be considered. In the clinical literature, particular psychotic symptoms suggest different etiologies; for example, visual hallucinations are common during alcohol withdrawal, whereas delusional parasitosis is more typical of stimulant intoxication. Delirious patients can exhibit a variety of psychoses, but they less frequently experience mania.

MOOD DISORDER SECONDARY TO MEDICAL ILLNESS AND MAJOR NEUROCOGNITIVE DISORDER DUE TO FRONTOTEMPORAL DEMENTIA

You continue to see Daniel in your outpatient clinic. Six months after Daniel's hospitalization, Samira calls you and reports, "My father is acting strange again." When Daniel comes to see you, he insists that he is in the middle of preparing to win a reality cooking show and become a world-famous chef. He has been staying up all night trying out new recipes and has spent nearly $20,000 on cookbooks in the past month. He is very energetic, is talking quickly, and becomes irritated whenever you try to interrupt him. On further questioning, Samira reports that Daniel had a head injury from a mechanical fall about 2 months ago and lost consciousness for a couple of minutes. He "appeared fine" by the time the emergency department doctor saw him and was sent home. You diagnose Daniel with manic symptoms secondary to traumatic brain injury (TBI). You conclude that he is gravely disabled by his condition and offer him psychiatric hospitalization. After he declines, you speak again with Samira, who says that she is unable to care for her father at home in his current state, so you reluctantly conclude that

Daniel requires involuntary hospitalization to treat his manic episode. He responds well to empiric treatment with valproic acid while you pursue a definitive cause. His initial serum and urine studies are unremarkable, and he refuses to lie still for brain magnetic resonance imaging (MRI), so you order a head computed tomography scan, which is also unremarkable. Daniel does well and is discharged home on valproic acid. At your recommendation, he takes the medication for a few months, before discontinuing the medication against your recommendation.

Samira brings Daniel back 3 months later because his behavior has worsened; he is even more disinhibited. In public, he interrupts strangers with non sequiturs. In private, he eats several family-size bags of chips each day. With Samira's encouragement, Daniel consents to a brain MRI, which shows moderate bilateral frontotemporal atrophy. You diagnose him with behavioral variant frontotemporal dementia and refer him to a geriatric psychiatrist and behavioral neurologist for further management.

Typically, the onset of mania among older adults in a medical or surgical setting can be attributed to a medication or other substance. Corticosteroid use, particularly during titration or taper, is associated with both manic and depressive symptoms. Antidepressants and light therapy can trigger substance-induced mania in susceptible individuals. Caffeine and stimulant intoxication can cause hypomanic or manic symptoms. In most cases, substance-induced manic symptoms resolve once the offending agent is discontinued or its withdrawal period ends. Still, it is prudent to follow a person over time to be certain of the diagnosis.

In an older adult, the development of mania or psychosis should initially raise suspicion of an undiagnosed medical or neurological disorder rather than a primary psychiatric disorder. The presentation of mania or psychosis as a primary psychiatric disorder typically occurs as the brain develops in adolescence or early adulthood, rather than as the brain declines with age. When an adult older than age 50 experiences mania or psychosis for the first time, the practitioner should do a workup for substances and medical or neurological causes, as outlined in Table 4–1, before diagnosing a bipolar disorder or schizophrenia.

For many older adults, the development of a neurological disorder is associated with their initial experience of manic or psychotic symptoms. In the literature, about 5%–10% of peo-

TABLE 4–1. Workup for new-onset manic or psychotic symptoms in older adults

Neurological examination (with a focus on soft neurological and frontal release signs)

Serum laboratory workup for potential medical or neurological causes

    Complete blood count

    Chemistries and electrolytes, including creatinine, calcium, and magnesium

    Liver function panel

    Thyroid-stimulating hormone and other thyroid tests as indicated

    Vitamin B_{12} and folate levels

    Heavy metal screen if clinically indicated

Urine workup for potential medical or neurological causes

    Urinanalysis

    Urine toxicology screen

Cognitive screen such as the Montreal Cognitive Assessment (MoCA)

Medication review (with a focus on temporal association with symptoms)

Neuroimaging, if clinically indicated

    Magnetic resonance imaging (MRI) is preferred to head computed tomography because of the increased anatomic resolution

    Positron emission tomography can be used if patient has contraindication to MRI or if MRI does not show any definitive findings consistent with a particular type of dementia

Electroencephalography, if clinically indicated, to evaluate for seizures

Cerebrospinal fluid (including beta amyloid and tau markers to measure for Alzheimer's disease and the 14-3-3 marker to measure for prion disease), if clinically indicated (Muayqil et al. 2012)

ple with Huntington's disease develop mania, and more than 10% have psychotic symptoms (Rosenblatt 2007). Up to 60% of people with Parkinson's disease can be affected by psychosis, especially as the disease progresses and as dopaminergic agents are prescribed to treat motor symptoms (Forsaa et al. 2010). Impulse-control symptoms, which can sometimes be similar to manic symptoms, affect about 13.6% of patients with Parkinson's disease (Weintraub et al. 2010). Less commonly, about 10% of patients with TBI develop mania or psychotic symptoms (Jorge 2015; Jorge et al. 1993; Shukla et al. 1987). Poststroke mania and poststroke psychosis are even rarer (Rabins et al. 1991; Santos et al. 2011). A careful history, including a thorough family history, can be quite helpful in the evaluation of potential neurological disorders.

As the case of Daniel illustrates, however, untangling the initial presentation of a neurological disorder from the first presentation of manic or psychotic symptoms can be difficult. Daniel's manic symptoms were originally thought to be from the TBI. Sometimes, however, practitioners can be misled by seemingly related events that turn out to be unrelated—such as a TBI causing cognitive difficulties and a spousal death causing depression—and an undiagnosed disorder sometimes takes time to declare itself. Manic symptoms can be associated with a TBI but usually self-resolve after a few months (Jorge et al. 1993). With Daniel, it eventually became clear that he had developed an undiagnosed neurodegenerative disorder. The diagnosis of early, atypical, rapidly progressive dementias, such as major neurocognitive disorder due to frontotemporal dementia, can be difficult to make because caregivers often describe behavioral rather than cognitive symptoms. In these challenging diagnostic situations, it may be beneficial to make a subspecialty referral. A geriatric psychiatrist or behavioral neurologist can help diagnose early-onset atypical dementias such as frontotemporal dementia and Huntington's disease, which can be identified around age 50 or even younger (Bang et al. 2015; Epping et al. 2016).

SCHIZOPHRENIA

Nowadays, more adults with schizophrenia are living to advanced age and in the community. In many cases, there is "positive aging" in schizophrenia, meaning that as some patients age, they have fewer positive psychotic symptoms such as hallucinations and require hospitalization less frequently. Many older patients with schizophrenia, however, continue to struggle with negative symptoms, such as cognitive problems, amotivation, and minimal social interaction. Slowly tapering off antipsychotics to geriatric-appropriate doses when clinically appropriate and removing anticholinergic medications used to manage extrapyramidal symptoms are important strategies for reducing the side effects from these medications, such as increased risk of metabolic syndrome, stroke, death, and cognitive impairment. See Chapter 16 ("Psychopharmacological Interventions") for more information about medication discontinuation.

SLEEP-RELATED HALLUCINATIONS AND VISUAL HALLUCINATIONS DUE TO VISUAL IMPAIRMENT

> Esther, a 91-year-old woman with stage 4 congestive heart failure and COPD who requires supplemental oxygen and is legally blind in her right eye because of macular degeneration, presents to your office concerned about auditory hallucinations. While falling asleep recently, she has been hearing the voices of people from her childhood who have died. You review her medication list, discontinue her zolpidem, and recommend sleep hygiene measures. On a subsequent visit, she reports that her auditory hallucinations have resolved but wonders if they are related to the strange visions she has experienced since she lost sight in her right eye. She sometimes sees small cats wandering around her house, even though she does not own any pets and knows the cats are not really there.

Hypnogogic (as a person is going to sleep) and hypnopompic (as a person is waking up) hallucinations are common and benign sleep-related hallucinations, occurring in about 25% of the population at some point in life (American Sleep Association 2007). Esther is additionally experiencing visual hallucinations secondary to blindness or impaired vision; these experiences, known as Charles Bonnet syndrome, generally require only education so that a patient understands that his mind is filling in complex images because of visual impairment. Reassurance and reality testing, which can be easily accomplished because most people do not experience accompanying auditory or tactile hallucinations, and distraction if the images are bothersome are usually all that is required (Menon et al. 2003).

DELUSIONAL DISORDER

The following winter, Esther is brought to the emergency department by a crisis management team because she has made multiple phone calls to 911 asking that her landlord be arrested. Esther believes he has been trying to poison her by releasing toxic fumes through her apartment's heating vents. After spending the night in the emergency department, she is discharged to a same-day appointment in your clinic. She tells you that about 6 months ago her landlord tried to evict her from her rent-controlled apartment so he could give it to another person who would pay full price. Although his attempt was unsuccessful, Esther became anxious that he would try to drive her out through other means. During your interview, you are unable to elicit other psychotic thoughts. A psychiatric review of systems and Esther's medical and neurological examinations are all unremarkable. Her score on the Mini-Mental State Examination (MMSE) is 29/30, and Esther denies any functional decline. She refuses any treatment but decides that fighting her landlord is interfering with her sleep and elects to move in with her daughter.

Three years later, Esther returns with her daughter and claims that her daughter has been replaced by an identical-appearing person. Esther's MMSE score is 29/30, and she continues to refuse treatment. She has no functional decline.

Delusional disorder is characterized by the experience of one or more delusions lasting at least 1 month. The prevalence of delusions in older adults without dementia is approximately 5%; the two main types are persecutory and misidentification (Holt and Albert 2006). Common persecutory delusions in older adults without dementia include thoughts of neighbors or landlords trying to evict them, property theft, abandonment, and jealousy of a spouse because of suspected but unproven infidelity. Misidentification delusions include misidentification of common people, which is known as a Capgras delusion; phantom boarder syndrome, in which patients believe there are noisy and disruptive strangers in the house; misidentification of objects; misidentification of self-image in the mirror; and misidentification of TV characters as being real. Practitioners can help patients like Esther by assessing for delusions and reality testing.

Mental Health Disorders Contributing to or Exacerbating Medical Disorders

Carla is a 66-year-old woman with poorly controlled hypertension and osteoporosis who was seen 10 times in the emergency department last year with episodes of hypertensive urgency. Although there are no apparent financial or cognitive barriers to taking medication, Carla consistently misses doses. When a pharmacist visits Carla's home, he finds half her pills untaken. Carla declines his offer of a timer to remind herself to take her pills as prescribed. Instead, she explains that she skips her antihypertensives because "I don't feel like taking them—I feel fine." When Carla visits your office, you diagnose her with psychological factors affecting other medical conditions. She is referred to a psychologist in an integrated primary care–mental health group who identifies several factors that limit Carla's engagement with treatment, including distrust of the medical profession, anxiety about unnecessary medications, and limited understanding of how blood pressure control can have positive long-term health effects.

Psychological factors affecting other medical conditions is included in the somatic symptom disorders chapter of DSM-5 (American Psychiatric Association 2013). The somatic symptom disorders were designed for the use of non–mental health practitioners because people with these disorders rarely present directly to mental health practitioners. Most patients with these disorders are so committed to understanding their symptoms medically that they are unlikely to seek mental health treatment. The new DSM-5 diagnosis of psychological factors affecting other medical conditions is especially helpful for primary care practitioners and other non–mental health subspecialists who have struggled to treat patients who are "noncompliant" or who exacerbate their medical conditions because of untreated mental health disorders. Referring these types of patients to mental health care can be quite tricky, so their treatment often occurs in primary care settings. When seeing these patients, non–mental health practitioners should 1) avoid unnecessary medical evaluations or surgical procedures and 2) integrate behavioral health into otherwise medicalized visits, either through their own interventions or through those of psychologists or other mental health professionals working in medical care settings.

When mental health practitioners are integrated into a setting, patients can easily be referred for stress reduction techniques such as learning how to incorporate lifestyle changes or cognitive-behavioral therapy without feeling the stigmatization of mental health treatment for a physical problem.

Sexual Dysfunction

Paul is a 71-year-old man with obesity, hypertension, and poorly controlled diabetes who complains of not being able to have sex with his wife anymore and feeling embarrassed about his lack of performance. "I tried that blue pill from my friend a few times, but it didn't work." For the past 5 years he has taken sertraline 200 mg/day for depression, and his mood symptoms are well controlled. He denies any other psychiatric symptoms. His medication list also includes temazepam for sleep, propranolol for hypertension, and metformin for diabetes.

Paul describes his problem as difficulty with getting an erection and taking longer to ejaculate. You diagnose him with medication-induced dysfunction but strongly suspect his lifestyle habits also contribute to his sexual dysfunction. First, you work with him to take brisk walks 30 minutes a day and stop smoking. Over the next 3 months, you decrease his sertraline to 100 mg/day, taper off the temazepam, and instruct him in sleep hygiene techniques. You refer him to a primary care mental health psychologist so he can set realistic expectations for sexual performance at his age, comply with a diabetic diet, and lose about 20 pounds. After making all of these changes, Paul reports significant improvement in his delay in ejaculation but still has some trouble with erections, so you refer him to a urologist for further evaluation.

A common misperception is that older adults are "asexual." In fact, sex is an important part of many older adults' lives (Kessel 2001). Unfortunately, many older adults are not as sexually active as they wish to be for a variety of reasons, including psychosocial (e.g., not having a partner, marital discord), physiological (e.g., complications from genitourinary surgeries, restrictions on physical activity after cardiothoracic surgery), psychiatric (e.g., depression, other untreated psychiatric disorders), and taking medically necessary drugs that affect sexual functioning.

Aggression and Agitation

Aggression and agitation are common problems of older adults with dementia whether they are living in their own homes, with relatives, or in institutional settings such as assisted living and skilled nursing facilities.

> Jose is a 72-year-old man who had a right middle cerebral artery infarction 2 months ago. Since his stroke he requires full care for his activities of daily living, and he is now brought in by his three daughters because he frequently kicks them when they try to bathe and change him at the end of the day.

Managing episodes of aggression and agitation in older adults can be challenging, particularly in those with dementia. Nonpharmacological approaches are considered to be first-line treatment for behavioral disturbances, including aggression and agitation. The DICE (**D**escribe, **I**nvestigate, **C**reate, and **E**valuate) model provides an evidence-based approach to managing neuropsychiatric symptoms of older adults with dementia (Kales et al. 2014) (Table 4–2).

> The practitioner realizes that Jose's daughters were taking him out all day while they ran errands and visited friends, then expected him to sit through an hour-long family dinner. By bedtime, Jose was exhausted and acting out. The key to figuring out that he was exhausted is that the three daughters, despite splitting their caregiving duties, were also very tired. When you are unsure why a patient is acting a certain way, remember this clinical maxim: "The caregiver's mood usually mirrors the patient's." Jose's daughters agree to send him to an adult day care center several days a week to enable them to accomplish their errands without taking him along. After they understand that the noise and chaos of children and grandchildren is overstimulating their father, they decide to let Jose eat quietly upstairs with one family member rather than join their large sit-down dinner every night. Jose is then able to feel calm and behave agreeably in the evening.

Self-Harm, Suicide, and End-of-Life Concerns

Practitioners, particularly those in mental health, are commonly presented with patients who hurt themselves, whether intentionally or not. To help you understand the

TABLE 4–2. DICE intervention

Step	Description
Describe	Caregivers are asked to **describe** in as much detail as possible the events leading up to the behavior, the behavior itself, and the resulting distress. Behavioral logs and videos can be helpful in pinpointing potential precipitants that lead up to the behavior.
Investigate	The practitioner **investigates** reasons for the behavioral disturbances, including untreated pain, medication side effects, disrupted sleep-wake cycles, sensory changes, environmental changes, and boredom or overstimulation.
Create	Patient, caregiver, and practitioner/team **collaboratively create** a plan of action. Collaboration with all caregivers is the key to successful creation and implementation of the plan. For example, learning about a patient's favorite activities can help keep him properly engaged or distracted to reduce agitation.
Evaluate	The practitioner **evaluates** whether the intervention was safe and effective. For example, has there been decreased frequency or intensity of the behavioral disturbance? If evaluation determines that the intervention was not safe or effective, the practitioner should go back and review the previous steps.

Source. Adapted from Kales et al. 2014.

scope of the problem, we present three scenarios that demonstrate the ways patients hurt themselves, through either intentional neglect or self-harm.

> Beth is a 76-year-old woman who has a body mass index of 42.0, binge-eating disorder, end-stage renal disease on hemodialysis, and poorly controlled diabetes. During rehabilitation in the hospital after hip and knee replacement surgery, she displays difficult behavior toward the staff, such as refusing insulin or rehabilitation unless she is given opiates to help with diabetic neuropathy and asking her friends to bring sweets from the outside. During her hospital stay, she develops nonhealing ulcers from lying in bed, which are worsened by her blood sugar frequently being in

Beyond the Diagnostic Ds

the 400s. When the team approaches her about intermittent compliance, she replies, "I don't care if I die from diabetes— I will eat whatever I want." The team dismisses her as a willful and difficult patient. Beth remains hospitalized when no facility will accept her because of her uncooperative behavior and need for hemodialysis. Two months later she becomes septic from an infected decubitus ulcer and dies. Her daughter, who was not involved in her mother's care until a week prior to death, sues the hospital for negligence because psychiatry was never consulted.

Darryl is a 91-year-old male with end-stage COPD, congestive heart failure with an ejection fraction of 20%, and stage 4 ulcers, whose children moved him into an assisted living facility 2 months ago. They bring him into the office because after he declared "I'm so sick that I cannot do anything—I might as well be dead," they discovered he was reading Web sites about suicide. Darryl is diagnosed with major depressive disorder and responds well to depression-focused psychotherapy. After an extensive discussion with a geriatric medicine consultant and a family meeting, his children agree to stop pushing their father to pursue aggressive care and agree to work with palliative care to improve his quality of life. Darryl dies about 1 year after you meet him. His children reach out to let you know that Darryl felt that palliative care helped him come to peace with his medical illness and he died comfortably.

Arnie is an 83-year-old man, recently widowed for the third time, referred for treatment of depression after he unexpectedly fired his home health services and refused assistance for instrumental activities of daily living. His first wife died unexpectedly of renal cancer; his second wife died from complications of diabetes; and his third wife died from terminal lung cancer 3 months after she was diagnosed. The patient, who adamantly denies any depressive symptoms or suicidality, reluctantly agrees to return for a follow-up visit but never comes. He is found at home, unconscious after overdosing on acetaminophen in the same bed where his wife died. A letter he wrote described recurring nightmares of seeing his wife die and expressed fear he might see someone else close to him succumb soon. Arnie is hospitalized and dies 2 days later from liver failure.

Adults age 85 and older have the second highest suicide rate among all age groups: 18.6 per 100,000 people in the United States in 2013 (American Foundation for Suicide Prevention 2015). Assessing suicidal risk by asking, "Are you suicidal?" is insufficient and inaccurate. Rather, an analysis of risk factors is necessary. Accurately predicting whether a patient will make a lethal suicide attempt is extremely difficult. The Web site of the Substance Abuse and Mental Health Services Administration (2015) has examples of suicide risk assessment. Practitioners should also consider creating a suicide safety plan for patients who engage in self-harm or are at high risk for suicide (Suicide Prevention Resource Center 2015). Components of a suicide safety plan include identification of protective factors, involvement of family, and modification of environmental factors (e.g., removal of firearms, placement of firearms in a gun safe, or use of a gun lock; locking up medications or using timed pill boxes so the patient cannot impulsively overdose). As demonstrated in all three of the above scenarios, a variety of mental health diagnoses can lead to self-neglect, self-harm, and suicide. The diagnoses in these cases include binge-eating disorder and probably undiagnosed personality and mood disorders in Beth; major depressive disorder and end-of-life concerns in Darryl; and untreated major depressive disorder after his wife's death in Arnie.

There are two steps to effectively managing self-neglect, self-harm, and suicidal behavior: 1) conducting a thorough psychiatric evaluation and 2) engaging a multidisciplinary team to address both physical and mental health components contributing to an older patient's suicidal thoughts. The team can include but is not limited to practitioners from primary care, relevant medical subspecialties, psychiatry, psychology, and palliative care. Psychiatry is important for pharmacological treatment of any mental health disorders, whereas psychology can help older adults as they physically and cognitively decline to achieve ego integrity and wisdom, improve distress tolerance, and resist despair (Kasl-Godley and Christie 2014). Palliative care helps patients feel comfortable and can alleviate wanting to die merely to relieve distress. Involvement of the caregiver or nursing manager in a structured setting is also important for behavioral management. In fact, as demonstrated in Beth's and Darryl's scenarios, failure to involve the caregiver when an older patient has a poor prognosis due to psychiatric and/or medical illness may lead to a poor patient outcome, as well as legal action.

CHAPTER 5

The 15-Minute Older Adult Diagnostic Interview

PERFORMING a 15-minute interview with an older adult experiencing mental distress sounds impossible. Older adults have a lifetime of stories to tell, as well as accrued ailments and impediments of age and, often, an inability to name them succinctly. Gathering the crucial information in only 15 minutes requires a skilled interviewer. As you are developing this skill, remember the purpose of a brief interview. You cannot generate a complete differential diagnosis and a comprehensive treatment plan in 15 minutes, but you can seek the most likely diagnoses, identify a psychiatric emergency such as suicidality or elder neglect, and initiate treatment. Consider the following case:

> Marcos, a 66-year-old man, presents to your primary care office to establish care. He tells your medical assistant that he "feels sad all the time." She asks him to complete a Patient Health Questionnaire 9-item depression scale (PHQ-9), Generalized Anxiety Disorder 7-Item Scale (GAD-7), and the DSM-5 Level 1 Cross-Cutting Symptom Measure prior to your 15-minute visit (American Psychiatric Association 2013). His scores for the PHQ-9 and GAD-7 are 12 and 10, respectively. On his DSM-5 Level 1 Cross-Cutting Symptom Measure, he indicates some concern about depression, anxiety, and alcohol use. Reading over these results, you may find yourself feeling pressured because there are so many concerns to cover in 15 minutes.

When meeting a patient like Marcos for a 15-minute interview, we rely on three key strategies:

1. Obtain as much background information as possible before the interview. Review any available records. Under-

stand, if possible, why the patient is visiting today and with whom. Review any validated mental health screenings a patient and/or her caregiver completed prior to the visit. These screenings, particularly the DSM-5 Level 1 Cross-Cutting Symptom Measure, can give an idea of where to initially focus your diagnostic questions.

2. Observe the patient's functional status during the interview. If possible, walk your patient to an examination room. This simple courtesy gives you an opportunity to observe how the patient dresses, greets a stranger, ambulates, and navigates a space outside of her own dwelling.

3. Determine whether the patient's functional status matches her current level of social support and care. Learning how well a patient's psychosocial needs and her currently available resources fit together is critical for deciding the first steps of your treatment plan. For example, a patient who is living independently without any significant social support but needs assistance with instrumental activities of daily living (IADLs) will have greater difficulty implementing your recommendations than one who is fully dependent on others for IADLs but benefits from a strong support network in an assisted living facility.

Outline of 15-Minute Older Adult Diagnostic Interview

MINUTE 1

Review the screening responses before meeting the patient. Formulate in your mind what areas you want to focus on and how you intend to structure your interview.

MINUTE 2

Introduce yourself and explain the length and purpose of today's interview.

MINUTES 3–6

Start with a general question (e.g., "Tell me, what brought you here?") or a more specific comment tied to the screening materials (e.g., "Tell me more about the depressive symptoms you have had recently"). Instead of asking a list of closed-ended questions, allow a patient to narrate the history of her present illness. Get a sense of how well the patient can organize her history, how long she has been experiencing these symptoms, and how they affect her daily routine.

MINUTES 7–10

If possible, collect collateral information from the patient's caregiver(s). If no caregiver is available, take these 3 minutes to do a psychiatric review of systems and a brief cognitive screening, which includes orientation and delayed recall.

MINUTES 11–12

Collect past psychiatric history and screen for red flags such as high risk for suicide, elder abuse, and heavy substance use, any of which will require you to refer your patient for further treatment, such as from mental health or social work practitioners. For the psychiatric history, determine whether or how long the person has been in mental health treatment; whether she has been hospitalized for psychiatric reasons; and whether there have been any suicide or homicide attempts and, if so, the lethality of those attempts. For the psychotropic history, you primarily need to know which antidepressants the patient has tried and whether she has ever taken a mood stabilizer and/or antipsychotic. You can speed up this process by having her review a list of psychotropic medications beforehand to check which ones have been previously prescribed.

MINUTES 13–15

By the end of the interview, you should know which of these actions is needed for your patient: 1) obtain further information and/or treat in primary care; 2) refer to mental health services for further treatment; or 3) in very rare circumstances, refer to emergency psychiatric services. Finally, you should share your initial treatment plan with the patient.

For example, the following is one way to structure a 15-minute interview with Marcos, the patient introduced at the beginning of this chapter.

> Minute 1: Introduce yourself and the purpose of today's conversation. "Hi, Mr. Pena. I'm Dr. Ryan, and today I'll be spending about 15 minutes to talk to you about your mental health."

Minute 2: Summarize the results of Marcos's screening questionnaires, beginning with his depressive and anxiety symptoms, followed by the potentially more sensitive subject of his alcohol use.

Minutes 3–6: Tell Marcos something like, "I see you indicated you were feeling depressed recently. Please tell me more about that." Because Marcos explains that he has been depressed and anxious for the past 3 months since being diagnosed with hepatitis C by his previous primary care practitioner, observe not just what he says but how he says it, listening for his emotional tone, cognitive ability, and character structure. Marcos tells you that he used heroin intravenously until about 30 years ago, when he enrolled in a methadone program; he has been abstinent ever since. He is embarrassed about his diagnosis and is anxious that his hepatologist will say he needs to go on a special regimen to treat his hepatitis C. He is also afraid to tell his family because he fears they will reject him.

Minutes 7–10: During the psychiatric review of systems, Marcos reports that he drinks 1–2 shots of tequila about 4–6 times per week after he gets home from work. Since his diagnosis of hepatitis C, he has also been drinking 1–2 beers per night to help him go to sleep. When you ask whether Marcos thinks he has a problem with drinking, he says he does not. However, he acknowledges that his hepatologist is concerned about his drinking.

Minutes 11–12: During your review of his history, Marcos denies any psychiatric history other than his treatment in the methadone clinic.

Minutes 13–15: During your final minutes, you begin by asking Marcos how interested he is in mental health treatment. He reports ambivalence about taking medication but agrees to discuss the stress of his new diagnosis of hepatitis C with the psychologist who is part of your clinic's new primary care–mental health integration initiative. Hoping to spark Marcos's interest in treatment, you use motivational interviewing techniques to prepare him for return visits and engagement in mental health treatment.

Handling Challenges in the 15-Minute Interview

OBTAINING THE PATIENT HISTORY

In an idealized world, when an older adult presents for her first mental health visit, she will start off with a chief complaint, tell a well-prepared story about her symptoms, and then eagerly adopt your treatment recommendations. In the real world, a patient's path to mental health assessment and treatment is frequently characterized by false starts, dead ends, and circuitous routes that often exasperate caregivers. The reasons are many: cost and access are prohibitive barriers in many communities, adverse experiences with mental health practitioners in the past keep many patients away, and many people have internalized stigma about mental illness despite little actual exposure to mental health treatment.

As we discussed in Chapter 1, "Introduction," when you are working with older adults who have internalized stigma about mental illness, it is essential to develop a strong therapeutic alliance in order to obtain an accurate history. Giving an older adult time to discuss her concerns can also be quite important, because it allows her to reveal important information about her own or a family member's history of mental illness. Even bringing up the topic of mental health for the first time can be challenging, especially during a short primary care visit. We usually introduce the question of mental health symptoms with an acknowledgment that such feelings of distress are common in the geriatric population. For example, we might say, "People often feel sad after a spouse has died. I'm wondering whether you are having such feelings since Mr. Locke died 2 months ago."

Another common barrier to obtaining a meaningful history is *alexithymia*, the inability to describe feelings using words. Sometimes, older adults deny any mental health issues despite having behaviors or informant reports that strongly suggest mental distress and even illness. Reasons for alexithymia are not always pathological—some generations and cultures do not encourage expressing one's feelings directly and, in fact, look down on expression of emotion as a weakness or character flaw. Nevertheless, common, vague answers such as "I'm fine" or "OK, I guess" can be frustrating for practitioners who sense deeper issues. Instead of asking direct, structured interview questions such as "What is your mood today?" or "Do you hear voices?" practitioners may be more successful asking older adults about daily routines, interests, and cultural background, using "what if" questions, such as "If your wife were alive, what would you be doing differently?" In some cultures, expressing mental distress as physical symptoms, such as stomach complaints or chronic pain, may be more socially acceptable. In these cases, practitioners should rate improvement on the basis of whatever culturally appropriate measures the patient feels comfortable reporting. For example, asking about changes in stomach pain may yield more information than direct questions about the patient's mood, which is reported as "always fine."

EXPLORING WHY PATIENTS REJECT HELP

During the treatment planning part of your 15-minute interview, Marcos explains that he does not want any medications for depression or anxiety at this time. "I'm already going to have to take medications for my liver problems. I don't think it would be good for my liver to take more." You may feel frustrated because although Marcos is disinterested in an antidepressant because of the possibility it will harm his liver, he is still drinking alcohol.

Older adults who appear to be rejecting mental health treatment can be challenging to treat, particularly for younger or inexperienced practitioners. It is important to remember that there are many reasons for help-rejecting behaviors. Some people refuse help because they have symptoms of a mental illness, such as feelings of worthlessness from untreated depression or the sense of superiority from narcissistic personality disorder. Some older patients reject help simply because they are unwilling to add an additional medication to an already lengthy medication list. Some worry about side effects, have had bad experiences from prescribed psychotropic medications, or know people who have experienced adverse effects. Others may be anxious about medical nightmares they have read about online. When a patient rejects help, you can seek the meaning of the rejection by gently pointing out her ambivalence: "You say that you want your depressive symptoms to get better, but then you tell me that you do not believe medications or therapy will help. I'm wondering whether you have something else in mind that may treat your depression, or if you have concerns about medications or therapy that we have not talked about."

Another possible reason for help-rejecting behavior is that a patient might not have a strong enough therapeutic alliance with you to trust your recommendations. If this appears to be the situation, it can help to explore the patient's misgivings about your treatment plan together or encourage her to discuss your treatment plan with another practitioner whom she trusts.

Treating the mental health conditions of older adults poses special challenges. Because at least 50% of depressed older patients do not fully respond to a first-line antidepressant, it is likely that many will need additional treatment such as depression-focused psychotherapy (Reynolds et al. 2010). Given this high likelihood of failure, it is important to build leeway into your therapeutic alliance; leeway allows you to "fail" while maintaining your therapeutic alliance. One common reason patients refuse to continue taking medications or do not return for follow-up mental health treatment is that they experience adverse effects and then blame a practitioner for being incompetent. You can anticipate this concern by setting realistic expectations for initial treatments while remaining optimistic about an eventual positive outcome. You might say, "Many patients respond well to the first antidepressant we try, but some do not. I suggest trying venlafaxine first to address both your pain and depression. If you do not respond or have adverse effects, then we will work together to figure out what the next step will be."

TALKING ABOUT THE FORBIDDEN THREE Ss: SEX, SUBSTANCE USE, AND SUICIDE

Some older patients may be embarrassed to bring up topics they feel are out of bounds, such as sex, substance use, and suicide. Practitioners must carefully plan ahead so they can maintain the therapeutic alliance while they obtain information about these important topics. Bringing up these subjects proactively, but gently, is usually a good approach. Practitioners can naturally bring up the question of sexual activity in the context of providing psychoeducation on related topics. For example, you can introduce sexual activity as a topic when discussing the sexual effects of selective serotonin reuptake inhibitors. You might start the conversation by saying, "I want to let you know that some patients experience problems with ejaculating or having erections after starting sertraline. If this happens to you, please let me know immediately. Difficulties with sex and intimacy can affect your quality of life, and we have many approaches for reducing sexual side effects." By bringing up this sensitive subject in a medical context, practitioners communicate to patients that sexual activity is an important aspect of their health. This approach also allows patients to decide whether to discuss the subject further (e.g., "Actually, now that you mention it, I've been having trouble with my sex life since I started that blood pressure medication").

Sometimes practitioners can be surprised about where the difficulties occur in an interview. You may feel awkward when you talk to Marcos about his alcohol use during the psychiatric review of systems, only to be surprised when he reports without hesitation how much he drinks. Then, when you start to feel comfortable discussing his alcohol consumption, your discomfort returns when he denies having an alcohol problem even though he acknowledges that his hepatologist told him to stop drinking because "my liver tests are really high." When you ask Marcos what he thinks about what the hepatologist said, he replies, "Well, alcohol is natural and safe; you can just buy it in the store. I'm not even sure I need those liver drugs—he's probably getting extra money from drug companies to give them out."

Substance use can be a difficult topic to broach because both practitioners and older patients labor under stereotypes. Each of us has been occasionally surprised to discover that a pleasant, mild-mannered elderly woman is drinking a bottle of wine every night to deal with her insomnia and anxiety. Similarly, many older adults who have substance use disorders, especially for prescribed benzodiazepines or opioids, do not see themselves as stereotypical substance users. They may feel offended when asked directly, "Do you use illicit drugs such as cocaine or heroin?" To address the possible tension that may arise, we usually introduce the topic of substance use under the broader topic of lifestyle choices: "I'm going to ask you some questions about your lifestyle and health habits." We begin with relatively benign topics such as physical activity and dietary habits before asking about tobacco and alcohol use. At this point, a practitioner who senses tension about these more difficult questions can introduce the topic with an empathetic explanation: "Sometimes patients tell me they have felt so stressed out or are in so much pain that they took a pill offered by a relative or a good friend. Or maybe they were upset at their doctor for not treating their pain or anxiety, and then found another doctor who would give them additional medications to help their suffering. I'm wondering whether you have had such an experience."

It is common for practitioners and patients to disagree about what constitutes safe levels of substance use. Practitioners often get angry and frustrated when a patient continues to engage in substance use even after the negative effects on her health have been clearly explained. In this situation, a highly effective technique known as motivational interviewing—a process designed to engage patients to pursue behavioral changes for a wide range of issues, including substance use—may be helpful. The main tenets of motivational interviewing are empathy for the patient, reflective thinking, rolling with the resistance, and motivating the patient to believe that she can change (Substance Abuse and Mental Health Services Administration 2012).

Finally, perhaps the most difficult topic to address during a brief interview is suicide. Bringing up "the suicide question" can feel awkward even for experienced psychiatrists, and we still feel anxious when we ask long-established patients about it. Nevertheless, this important issue cannot be ignored, especially because people age 85 and older had the second-highest suicide rate (18.6 per 100,000) in the United States in 2013 (American Foundation for Suicide Prevention 2015). A strong therapeutic alliance is the key to feeling comfortable when asking the suicide question. Even though primary care practitioners might prefer deferring to mental health practitioners, studies indicate that the former are more likely to have contact with a patient prior to a suicide attempt (McDowell et al. 2011). Primary care providers play a critical role in suicide prevention, and the Prevention of Suicide in Primary Care Elderly: Collaborative Trial (PROSPECT) and Improving Mood-Promoting Access to Collaborative Treatment (IMPACT) clinical trials have demonstrated the importance of collaborative care between primary care and mental health providers to reduce suicidal ideation in the primary care setting (Bruce et al. 2004; Unützer et al. 2006).

Practitioners can reduce the stigma of suicide by educating patients about the benefits of disclosing suicidal thoughts and self-harm behaviors, reassuring patients that they are not "going crazy" when they express their thoughts of death and suicide, and exploring fears about what will happen if patients do bring up such thoughts. Useful cues for broaching the suicide question include the following: "Talking about your suicidal thoughts can help lower stress levels and makes it less likely that you will hurt yourself." "When people your age lose friends and family members, they sometimes start to think about their own death. Have you had any such thoughts recently?" "Sometimes people worry about what will happen to them if they tell me they have suicidal ideas—such as getting locked up. Do you have any such worries?" "I understand it can be difficult to talk about, but many of my other patients who have been through similar difficult experiences often have these thoughts. I want to reassure you that I do not think you are going crazy."

Obtaining an accurate answer to the suicide question can seem even more challenging. A recently widowed, kind-hearted patient once told one of us, "I would never kill myself, and I promise to make our next appointment in 4 weeks." Yet 2 weeks later he mailed a beautiful thank you card apologizing that he was planning to kill himself and would miss the appointment. After canceling the appointment, he overdosed on aspirin. Fortunately, he survived and, at a later visit, explained that "I did not want to upset you. I just did not want you to be worrying about someone as worthless as me." Moments like these remind us how the therapeutic relationship can cut both ways: patients feel the weight of our expectations just as much as we fear for their well-being.

Many practitioners fear that a patient who intends to kill herself will not disclose the truth or may change her mind after leaving the office and then make a serious attempt. To maximize the likelihood of getting an honest answer to safety questions, we approach suicide like any other mental health symptom. We encourage patients to talk about unsafe thoughts, rather than immediately ending the conversation with a referral to emergency services. Many patients have had suicidal thoughts for an extended period of time but only gradually find the courage to discuss them. Positive feedback such as "This is a really difficult topic—I'm glad you feel comfortable enough to share your thoughts with me" can help patients feel more bonded with their practitioner and less likely to hurt themselves by the end of the conversation. Most importantly, all patients, even those experiencing psychosis, want to be reassured that they are "not going crazy" by talking about suicidality and can get better. When they are able to express their thoughts about suicide openly, they will often feel less distressed about their symptoms and thus less likely to act rashly.

TIPS FOR THE 15-MINUTE INTERVIEW

Focus on broad brushstrokes rather than details.

Ask the older patient or informant to complete questionnaires or detailed intake packets before the interview to save time.

Make sure to ask about suicidality, homicidality, and substance use.

The best predictor of a future suicide attempt is a past suicide attempt. Consider the means for suicide currently available, the last time an attempt was made, and the number and lethality of previous attempts.

The best predictor of a future homicidal attempt is a past homicidal attempt. Consider the means currently available, the last time an attempt was made, and the number and lethality of previous attempts.

Offer options during treatment planning sessions (e.g., medications, psychotherapy, or both). This will help you gauge more accurately what treatment your patient feels ready to accept.

CHAPTER 6

The 30-Minute Older Adult Diagnostic Interview

AS busy practitioners, we sometimes forget the importance of making (and taking) moments to get to know our older patients beyond their answers to diagnostic questions. Sometimes we need to comfort a crying widower or chat about hobbies with a bluff retiree before we ask any diagnostic questions. In moments such as these, we may feel that we do not know what we are accomplishing in a conversation. We may desire to refocus the conversation because we have other people to see and other tasks to complete. Good interviewers, however, understand that these seemingly wasted moments are as integral to the interview. These moments are valuable for providing clues about whether the patient's distress is internal or external, what events bring him into and out of engagement with a practitioner, and how he formulates thoughts.

In an initial encounter, we start by getting to know the individual we are seeing. We use different strategies based on a person's functional ability, the location in which we are meeting, our familiarity with the patient, the patient's sense of humor, and any number of other variables. Before introducing ourselves to a patient, we like to know how long the patient has been waiting and with whom. The same patient will likely have different needs if he has sat calmly for 15 minutes in a waiting room than if he and his caregivers have been waiting hours in the emergency department. When we meet a person, we always prefer to open the conversation with a topic in which the person is already engaged. If he brings a book, we ask what it is about. If he is wearing the logo of a sports team, we ask about the team's most recent season. The point is not to make an aesthetic judgment about the patient's books or clothes but to understand how he thinks.

Asking about something that the patient is consciously (or unconsciously) presenting to you also builds the therapeutic alliance. Imagine if you walked into a medical encounter and your physician talked entirely about his interests while disregarding your attempts to discuss your own interests. You would most likely feel ignored and be reluctant to engage in treatment with the physician. Now imagine if you visited another physician and he knew your name, said it correctly, and then asked how you came by your name. You would likely be more responsive to this second physician and his treatment. You can (and should) extend the same engaging courtesy to the older adults you meet as patients.

We favor beginning every interview by introducing ourselves, asking an elder his name, assessing his expectations for the encounter, clarifying any misperceptions, and giving a sense of how long the encounter will last. We also like to know who arranged the visit: the person himself, his caregivers, or another practitioner. When someone else arranged for the evaluation, we acknowledge this immediately (e.g., "So your daughter wanted you to see me...") to show an older adult we can see things through his eyes.

Even if the encounter is limited to 30 minutes, we believe that you can successfully develop a therapeutic alliance and perform a diagnostic interview. Before we explain how, we offer a few caveats.

- Any psychiatric examination in which all the information comes from a single source is incomplete. This is especially true when interviewing older adults, who often depend on others. Ask the patient whom he relies on and seek his permission to discuss his health with that person. See Chapter 11, "Selected DSM-5 Assessment Measures," for tools to use in interviewing caregivers.

- A successful psychiatric examination ultimately provides access to the internal world of a person. The thoughts, impulses, and desires of an older person can be discovered in many ways. In what follows, we offer an interview that is best suited for a person who can tolerate direct questions. When interviewing someone who cannot do so because of age, impairment, or disinterest, we recommend focusing on the most essential portion of the examination and spending the remainder of your time developing a therapeutic alliance.

- A skilled psychiatric examination always includes an account of the relationships that constitute a person's existence. During every interview we ask questions such as these: "Whom do you live with?" "How do you spend your days?" "Who cares for you?" and "Whom can you trust?" These naturally open onto other critical questions about the caregivers in an elder's life.

With these caveats in mind, we offer the following as a guideline for a 30-minute diagnostic interview using DSM-5 criteria (American Psychiatric Association 2013). The interview does not include prompts for DSM-5 categories that are uncommon among older adults—namely, the neurodevelopmental, elimination, and paraphilic disorders. We have taught a version of this interview to students, residents, fellows, and faculty. Until you develop the habits of an experienced practitioner, it is useful to practice a structured interview. This practice helps in becoming comfortable asking about intimate concerns, remembering to screen all patients for the major categories of mental illness, and developing good interview habits.

Of course, using a structured interview has a downside. We have sometimes witnessed practitioners read one question after another, without stopping for the usual pauses that signify human speech or even looking at their patient. In the *Pocket Guide to the DSM-5 Diagnostic Exam* (Nussbaum 2013), these kinds of interviewers were called "psychiatric robots." They push along their agenda, saying, "I hear you are suicidal," but then before the patient can answer, they ask, "But do you really want to kill yourself now? And you don't really want to hurt anyone else, right?" Such questions demonstrate a focus on using the structured interview as a checklist rather than as a guide to asking probing questions in pursuit of understanding the person. Although relying on a checklist is important to making sure you have covered important topics, you should not rely on checklist interviewing as the only skill in your interview toolbox. To help you learn how to do the diagnostic interview, we will share with you other skills you need in your toolbox to successfully interview older adults.

Providing the right amount of structure for the interview is challenging. An excitable person will need to be soothed, a sad person will need to be encouraged, and sometimes one person will need both in the same interview. Fortunately, you always have the best possible guide: the person before you.

Follow his lead. Observe his body language. If he appears disinterested, it is time to alter your approach.

As you use this diagnostic interview, we recommend practicing a formal version until it becomes a habit and you develop a version that fits these questions to your own style and setting. The 30-minute diagnostic interview will seem forced at first, but gradually it provides the structure for a conversational interview.

Good interviewers always give a person a few minutes to speak his own mind. Then, after summarizing and clarifying his concern, they organize the examination as necessary, modulating the structure and language of the interview to fit the needs of the patient before them. They ask clear and succinct questions. If the patient is vague, they seek precision; if he remains vague, they explore why. They do not ask permission to change the subject but rather use transition statements, such as "I think I understand about [this], but how about [that]?" Developing a supply of stock questions is helpful, which is why we advise using this structured interview until it becomes a habit. These questions will help you develop a conversational interview in which a patient tells his story and you form an alliance with him, gain insight into his thought process, and gather the clinical data you need to make an accurate diagnosis. Developing a flow of exchange to the interview is important in building a therapeutic alliance.

Outline of the 30-Minute Older Adult Diagnostic Interview

The interview outline below includes headings that indicate the time allotted, instructions to the interviewer (roman type), and questions for the interviewer to ask (italic type).

MINUTE 1

Introduce yourself to the patient. Ask how he would like to be addressed. Set expectations for how long you will meet and what you will accomplish. Then say, *Tell me what brings you here today.*

MINUTES 2–4

Listen and observe. A patient's uninterrupted speech indicates much of his mental status, guides your history taking, and builds the alliance. As he speaks, notice both the content and the form of his statements. What is he saying, and how is he saying it? What is he not saying? How do his statements match his appearance? Although you may be tempted to interrupt or begin asking questions, with experience, you will find that allowing the person to talk initially without interruptions gives you more information about him than the answers to your questions will provide. When you do speak, try to have your next question be both responsive and open ended, such as *You said ____; can you tell me more about that?* Depending on the nature of the illness, some people will be unable to respond; their inability to do so also reveals valuable information about their mental status and distress. When the person does not speak spontaneously, you may have to use prompts and proceed to the history of present illness.

MINUTES 5–12

HISTORY OF PRESENT ILLNESS

Your questions should follow the DSM-5 criteria, as described in Chapter 7, "The DSM-5 Older Adult Diagnostic Interview." Additionally, you should focus on what has changed recently—the "why now?" of the presentation. As you do, seek understanding of precipitating events and make sure you can answer these questions: When did the patient's current distress begin? When was the last time he felt emotionally well? Can he identify any precipitating, perpetuating, or extenuating events? How have his thoughts and behaviors affected his psychosocial functioning? How does he view his current level of functioning, and how is it different from days, weeks, or months ago?

PAST PSYCHIATRIC HISTORY

When did you first notice symptoms? When did you first seek treatment? Did you ever experience a full recovery? Have you ever been hospitalized? How many times? What was the reason for those hospitalizations, and how long were you hospitalized? Do you receive outpatient mental health treatment? Do you take medications for a mental illness? Which medicines have helped the most? Did you experience adverse effects from any medications? What was the reason for stopping prior medications? How long were you taking each medication, and how often did you take it? Do you know the name, strength, and number of doses per day of medicines you're currently

*taking, including over-the-counter and herbal medicines? Have you
ever received injectable medications or electroconvulsive therapy?*

SAFETY

Students and trainees might feel uncomfortable asking safety
questions or worry that the questions might upset patients or
even give them ideas about ways to hurt themselves or others. These fears are largely unfounded, and with practice you
will find that these questions become much easier to ask. It is
important to remember that one of the biggest predictors of
future behavior is past behavior, so asking about prior episodes of violence to self and others is required for an overall
risk assessment.

*Do you frequently think about hurting yourself? Have you ever
hurt yourself, such as by cutting or hitting? Have you ever attempted to kill yourself? How many attempts have you made? What
did you do? What medical or psychiatric treatment did you receive
after these attempts? Do you often become so upset that you make
threats to hurt other people, animals, or property? Have you ever intentionally hurt people or animals, destroyed property, tricked other
people, or stolen things?* (See "Disruptive, Impulse-Control,
and Conduct Disorders" in Chapter 7.)

MINUTES 13–17

REVIEW OF SYSTEMS

The psychiatric review of systems is an overview of common
psychiatric symptoms that you may not have elicited in the
history of present illness. If a person answers yes to these
questions, you should explore further using the DSM-5 criteria, as modeled in Chapter 7.

Mood. *Have you been feeling sad, blue, down, depressed, or irritable?* If so: *Does feeling this way make it hard to do things, hard
to concentrate, or difficult to sleep? Has there been a time when for
many days in a row your mood was super happy, you were more
self-confident, and you had much more energy than usual?* If so:
Can you describe what happened? (See "Depressive Disorders"
or "Bipolar and Related Disorders" in Chapter 7.)

Psychosis. *Have you seen visions or other things that other people did not see? Have you heard noises, sounds, or voices that other
people did not hear? Do you ever feel as if people are following you
or trying to hurt you in some way? Have you ever felt that you had*

special powers or found special messages from the radio or TV that were seemingly meant just for you? (See "Schizophrenia Spectrum and Other Psychotic Disorders" in Chapter 7.)

Anxiety. *During the past several months, have you frequently been worried about a number of things in your life? Is it hard for you to control or stop your worrying? Are there specific things, places, or situations that make you feel very anxious or tearful? Have you ever felt suddenly frightened, nervous, or anxious for no reason at all?* (See "Anxiety Disorders" in Chapter 7.)

Obsessions and compulsions. *Do you ever get unwanted thoughts, urges, or pictures stuck in your mind that repeat, and you cannot make them stop? Is there anything you feel you have to check, clean, or organize over and over again in order to feel OK?* (See "Obsessive-Compulsive and Related Disorders" in Chapter 7.)

Trauma. *What is the worst thing that has ever happened to you? Has someone ever touched you in a way you did not want? Have you ever felt that your life was in danger or thought that you were going to be seriously injured? Do you have unhappy memories that make it hard to sleep or to feel OK now?* (See "Trauma- and Stressor-Related Disorders" in Chapter 7.)

Dissociation. *Everyone has trouble remembering things sometimes, but do you ever lose time, forget important details about yourself, or find evidence that you took part in events that you cannot recall? Do you ever feel as if people or places that are familiar to you are unreal? Do you ever feel as if you are standing outside your body or watching yourself? Do you lose track of time and feel unsure of what you did during that time?* (See "Dissociative Disorders" in Chapter 7.)

Somatic concerns. *Do you worry about your health more than most people? Do you get sick with aches and pains more often than most people your age do?* (See "Somatic Symptom and Related Disorders" in Chapter 7.)

Feeding and eating. *What do you think of your appearance? Do you ever restrict or avoid particular foods so much that your health or weight is negatively affected?* (See "Feeding and Eating Disorders" in Chapter 7.)

Sleeping. *Is your sleep often inadequate or of poor quality? Alternatively, do you often experience excessive sleepiness? Have you, or someone else, noticed any unusual behaviors while you sleep? Have* you, or someone else, noticed that you stop breathing or gasp for air while sleeping? (See "Sleep-Wake Disorders" in Chapter 7.)

Substance and other addictions.   How often do you drink alcohol? On the average day when you have at least one drink, how many drinks do you have? Have you had any problems as a result of drinking? When you stop drinking, do you go through withdrawal? Repeat for illicit and prescription drugs; begin by asking: Have you ever experimented with drugs? After asking about drugs, ask: Do you bet, wager, or gamble in a way that interferes with your life? (See "Substance-Related and Addictive Disorders" in Chapter 7.)

Personality.   When people reflect on their life, they can often identify patterns—characteristic thoughts, moods, and actions—that began when they were young and have since continued to occur in many personal and social situations. Thinking about your own life, can you identify any such patterns that have caused significant problems with your friends or family, at work, or in another setting? (See "Personality Disorders" in Chapter 7.)

MINUTES 18–23

PAST MEDICAL HISTORY

Do you have any chronic medical problems? Have these illnesses affected you emotionally? Have you ever undergone surgery? Have you ever experienced a seizure or hit your head so hard you lost consciousness? Do you take any medications for medical illness? Do you take any supplements, vitamins, over-the-counter medicines, or herbal supplements regularly?

Allergies.   Are you allergic to any medications? Can you describe your allergy?

Family history.   Have any of your relatives ever had mental or behavioral health problems, such as attention-deficit/hyperactivity disorder, anxiety, depression, bipolar disorder, psychosis, problems from drinking or drugs, suicide attempts, nervous breakdowns, or psychiatric hospitalizations?

Developmental history.   Do you know if your mother had any difficulties during her pregnancy or delivery? What were you like as a young child?

Social history.   Did you have any behavior or learning problems during your early childhood? How far did you go in school? Have *you ever served in the military? If so: For how long, and what rank and discharge did you achieve? How have you supported yourself? Currently? Was a religious faith part of your upbringing? Currently? Have you ever been arrested? Jailed? Imprisoned? What do you like to do? How do you spend your time online? What do you like about yourself? What do your friends like about you? Do you have any confidants? Are you sexually active? Have you been less interested in sex than usual or experienced difficulties in sexual performance?* (See "Sexual Dysfunctions" in Chapter 7.) *Are you really uncomfortable with your assigned gender?* (See "Gender Dysphoria" in Chapter 7.) *Do you feel safe in your current relationship? Are you, or have you been, married? Do you have any children? Grandchildren?*

MINUTES 24–28

MENTAL STATUS EXAMINATION

By this point in the interview, you should have already observed or obtained most of the pertinent mental status examination data. See Chapter 10, "The Mental Status Examination: A Psychiatric Glossary," for a more detailed version of the mental status examination, which includes the following components:

- Appearance
- Behavior
- Speech
- Emotion
- Thought process
- Thought content
- Cognition and intellectual resources
- Insight/judgment

MINI-MENTAL STATE EXAMINATION

The Mini-Mental State Examination (MMSE; Folstein et al. 1975) is a commonly used basic cognitive ability assessment used with older adults. It has standardized questions and yields a numerical score. These are useful lead-in questions: *Have you had any problems with your concentration or memory? Can you help me understand the extent to which you might be having those types of difficulty?* The MMSE includes the following items: name, date and time, place, immediate recall, attention (counting backward from 100 by 7s, spelling *world* back-

ward), delayed recall, general information (president, gover-
nor, five large cities), abstractions, proverbs, naming,
repetition, three-stage command, reading, copying, and writing. Scores below 24 (out of 30 points) indicate three levels of
cognitive impairment: mild (19–23 points), moderate (10–18
points), and severe (≤9). (See "Neurocognitive Disorders" in
Chapter 7.)

MINUTES 29–30

Ask any follow-up questions and quickly review your checklist to make sure you have covered all the important topics.
Thank the patient for his time and, if appropriate, begin discussing diagnosis and treatment.

Consider asking the following: *Have the questions I asked
addressed your major concerns? Is there anything important I
missed or anything that I really should know about to better understand what you are going through?*

SECTION II

Using DSM-5 With Older Adults

The DSM-5 Older Adult Diagnostic Interview

IN Chapter 6, "The 30-Minute Older Adult Diagnostic Interview," we outlined a diagnostic interview that includes questions to screen for each of the DSM-5 (American Psychiatric Association 2013) categories of mental disorders commonly experienced by older adults. When an older person answers affirmatively to one of those screening questions, the question should become the pathway into the psychiatric diagnostic interview. A good interviewer skillfully travels this path with an older person and, when possible, reaches a specific and accurate diagnosis along the way.

This chapter follows the order of DSM-5 disorder categories, beginning with schizophrenia spectrum and other psychotic disorders. For each category of DSM-5 diagnoses presented, the section begins with one or more screening questions from the model interview presented in Chapter 6 and then presents follow-up questions. If the follow-up questions include a measure of impairment or a measure of time, these measures are a required part of the subsequent diagnostic criteria. By asking follow-up questions before the additional symptom questions in the diagnostic criteria, we make the interview more efficient and precise while reserving the full diagnosis of a mental disorder until later.

The screening and follow-up questions are followed by the diagnostic criteria. When the diagnostic criteria are to be elicited by the interviewer, we offer italicized prompts for the relevant symptom. We structured these questions so that an affirmative answer meets the criteria for that symptom. When the diagnostic criteria are observed rather than elicited, as in the case of disorganized speech, psychomotor retardation, or autonomic hyperactivity, they are listed as instructions to the interviewer, set in roman type. The minimum number of symptoms necessary to reach a particular diagnosis is under-lined. We do not list all the possible questions that can be used to elicit a relevant symptom, but the included questions are specifically designed to follow DSM-5. To make the diagnostic process as clear as possible, we have included negative criteria for a DSM-5 diagnosis under the heading "Exclusion(s)." For example, DSM-5 observes that a person's avoidance of food to the point of significant weight loss does not meet criteria for avoidant/restrictive food intake disorder if it is better explained by food insecurity or a cultural practice such as fasting. These exclusion criteria usually do not require you to ask a specific question but instead depend on the history you elicit. The most common subtypes, specifiers, and severity measures are listed under the heading "Modifiers"; however, the complete array of modifiers is found only in DSM-5.

In the interest of brevity, this guide includes diagnostic questions for the most common DSM-5 disorders. The idea is to focus on learning diagnostic criteria for the most common disorders in each section before exploring the related diagnoses—that is, to know the main streets of DSM-5 before learning its side streets.

In this book, the side streets are labeled as *alternatives*, a term that is not used in DSM-5. These alternatives include only related diagnoses from the same DSM-5 diagnostic class. For example, schizophreniform disorder is listed as an alternative to schizophrenia because both are grouped in the same chapter in DSM-5. In contrast, major depressive disorder, obsessive-compulsive disorder, and some other diagnoses listed in the DSM-5 differential diagnosis for schizophrenia are not among the alternatives for schizophrenia listed in this chapter because they are in different diagnostic classes in DSM-5. For each diagnosis listed as an alternative, the essential criteria are included, and the interviewer is referred to the corresponding pages in DSM-5 to read the diagnostic criteria and associated material in detail.

We eliminated repetitive DSM-5 criteria, especially for the various mental disorders associated with another medical condition or substance-induced mental disorders, in which, broadly, the symptoms of a disorder are present as a direct effect of another medical condition or the use of a substance.

As this overview suggests, this book is not a substitute for DSM-5. It is a practical diagnostic tool that serves as an operationalized version of DSM-5—the equivalent of the sketched version of a city street that a satellite navigation device displays rather than the detailed portrait of each side street. If you need those details, use the letter and series of numbers that follow a diagnosis to direct you to additional information. For example, after gambling disorder, you will see this notation: [F63.0, 585–589]. The first entry is the ICD-10-CM code corresponding to gambling disorder, and the second entry is the page numbers of the main DSM-5 text for the disorder. These codes and page numbers are provided to assist practitioners with coding and with quickly locating additional information.

Unfortunately, the notations are sometimes more cryptic, as in this notation: [G47.4xx, 372–378]. As before, the first entry is the ICD-10-CM code corresponding to narcolepsy, and the second entry is the page numbers for the DSM-5 text about the disorder. However, the use of "xx" indicates that you need additional information to find the specific ICD-10-CM code. In this case, that additional information is whether a person's sleep disturbance occurs with or without cataplexy, hypocretin deficiency, or a genetic syndrome, or secondarily to another medical condition. We organized the diagnoses this way to reduce repetitive listing and keep your focus on efficient, accurate diagnoses.

ICD-10-CM codes are complex. Listing every code would double the length of this book and reduce its clinical utility. Listing every code would also shift the focus to accurate coding, when our goal is to help you make an accurate diagnosis as part of understanding another person.

As this strategy suggests, we try to balance brevity and detail. For each diagnosis, the notation always provides the general form of the ICD-10-CM codes along with the page numbers of DSM-5 so that you can quickly find the additional information you need. This book lacks the rich detail of DSM-5 but will deliver you to your diagnostic destination in a timely fashion.

Schizophrenia Spectrum and Other Psychotic Disorders

DSM-5 pp. 87–122

Screening questions: *Have you seen visions or other things that other people did not see? Have you heard noises, sounds, or* *voices that other people did not hear? Do you ever feel as if people are following you or trying to hurt you in some way? Have you ever felt that you had special powers or found special messages from the radio or TV that were seemingly meant just for you?*

If yes, ask: *Do these experiences change what you do or tell you to do things? Did these experiences ever cause you significant trouble with your friends or family, at work, or in another setting?*

- If yes, proceed to schizophrenia criteria.

1. Schizophrenia [F20.9, 99–105]

   a. Inclusion: Requires at least 6 months of continuous signs of disturbance, which may include prodromal or residual symptoms. During at least 1 month of that period, at least <u>two</u> of the following symptoms are present, and at least <u>one</u> of these symptoms must be delusions, hallucinations, or disorganized speech.

      i. Delusions: *Is anyone working to harm or hurt you? When you read a book, watch television, or work at a computer, do you ever find that there are messages intended just for you? Do you have special powers or abilities?*

      ii. Hallucinations: *When you are awake, do you ever hear a voice different from your own thoughts that other people cannot hear? When you are awake, do you ever see things that other people cannot see?*

      iii. Disorganized speech such as frequent derailment or incoherence

      iv. Grossly disorganized or catatonic behavior

      v. Negative symptoms such as diminished emotional expression or avolition

   b. Exclusion: If the disturbance is attributable to the physiological effects of a substance (e.g., a drug of abuse, a medication) or another medical condition, do not use this diagnosis.

   c. Modifiers

      i. Specifiers

         - First episode, currently in acute episode
         - First episode, currently in partial remission
         - First episode, currently in full remission
         - Multiple episodes, currently in acute episode

- Multiple episodes, currently in partial remission
- Multiple episodes, currently in full remission
- Continuous
- Unspecified

ii. Additional specifiers
- With catatonia [F06.1, 119–121]: At least <u>three</u> of the following are present: stupor, catalepsy, waxy flexibility, mutism, negativism, posturing, mannerisms, stereotypies, agitation, grimacing, echolalia, echopraxia.

iii. Severity
- Severity is rated by a quantitative assessment of the primary symptoms of psychosis, each of which may be rated for its current severity on a five-point scale (see "Clinician-Rated Dimensions of Psychosis Symptom Severity," DSM-5 pp. 742–744).

d. Alternatives

i. If a person has eccentric behaviors, perceptions, and thoughts, along with limited capacity for close relationships since early adulthood, consider schizotypal personality disorder [F21, 655–659]. If the disturbance occurs exclusively in the context of schizophrenia, a depressive or manic episode with psychotic features, or autism spectrum disorder, do not use this diagnosis.

ii. If a person experiences only delusions, whether bizarre or nonbizarre, has never met full criteria for schizophrenia, and has functioning that is not markedly impaired beyond the ramifications of her delusion, consider delusional disorder [F22, 90–93]. The criteria include multiple specifiers. Do not use this diagnosis if the delusions are due to the physiological effects of a substance or another medical condition. The diagnosis also should not be used if the delusions are better explained by another mental disorder.

iii. If a person has experienced at least 1 day but less than 1 month of schizophrenia symptoms, consider brief psychotic disorder [F23, 94–96]. The person usually has an acute onset of symptoms, exhibits fewer negative symptoms and less functional im-

pairment, and always experiences an eventual return to her previous level of functioning.

iv. If a person has experienced at least 1 month but less
than 6 months of schizophrenia symptoms, consider schizophreniform disorder [F20.81, 96–99].
The criteria include specifiers for catatonia, as well
as with and without good prognostic features.

v. If a person who meets criteria for schizophrenia also
experiences major mood disturbances—either major
depressive episodes or manic episodes—for at least
half the time she has met criteria for schizophrenia,
consider schizoaffective disorder [F25.x, 105–110].
Over a person's lifetime, she also must have experienced at least 2 weeks of delusions or hallucinations
in the absence of a major mood episode.

vi. If a substance or medication directly causes a psychotic episode, consider substance/medication-
induced psychotic disorder [F1x.x, 110–115].

vii. If another medical condition directly causes the
psychotic episode, consider psychotic disorder
due to another medical condition [F06.x, 115–118].

viii. If a person experiences psychotic symptoms that
cause clinically significant distress or functional
impairment without meeting full criteria for another psychotic disorder, consider unspecified
schizophrenia spectrum and other psychotic disorder [F29, 122]. If you wish to communicate the
specific reason a person's symptoms do not meet
the criteria, consider other specified schizophrenia spectrum and other psychotic disorder [F28,
122]. Examples include persistent auditory hallucinations in the absence of any other psychotic
symptom and delusional symptoms in the partner
of an individual with delusional disorder.

Bipolar and Related Disorders

DSM-5 pp. 123–154

Screening question: *Has there been a time when for many days
in a row your mood was super happy, you were more self-confident,
and you had much more energy than usual?*

If yes, ask: *During those times, did you feel this way all day or most of the day? Did something happen that started those feelings? Did those times ever last at least a week or result in your being hospitalized? Did these periods ever cause you significant trouble with your friends or family, at work, or in another setting?*

- If symptoms lasted a week or caused hospitalization, proceed to bipolar I disorder criteria.
- If not, proceed to bipolar II disorder criteria.

1. Bipolar I Disorder [F31.x, 123–132]
   For a diagnosis of bipolar I disorder, it is necessary to meet criteria for at least one manic episode. The manic episode may have been preceded by and may be followed by hypomanic episodes or major depressive episodes.

   a. Inclusion: A manic episode—defined as a distinct period of abnormally and persistently elevated or irritable mood and increased goal-directed activity or energy, lasting at least 1 week and present most of the day—requires at least <u>three</u> of the following symptoms.

      i. Inflated self-esteem or grandiosity: *During that period, did you feel especially confident, as though you could accomplish something extraordinary that you could not have done otherwise?*

      ii. Decreased need for sleep: *During that period, did you notice any change in how much sleep you needed to feel rested? Did you feel rested after less than 3 hours of sleep?*

      iii. More talkative than usual: *During that period, did anyone tell you that you talked more than usual or that it was hard to interrupt you?*

      iv. Flight of ideas: *During that period, were your thoughts racing? Did you have so many ideas that you could not keep up with them?*

      v. Distractibility: *During that period, were you having more trouble than usual focusing? Did you find yourself easily distracted?*

      vi. Increased goal-directed activity: *During that period, how did you spend your time? Did you find yourself much more active than usual?*

      vii. Excessive involvement in activities that have a high potential for painful consequences: *During that period, did you engage in activities that were unusual for you? Did you spend money, use substances, or engage in sexual activities in a way that is unusual for you? Did any of these activities cause trouble for anyone?*

b. Exclusions

    i. The occurrence of manic or major depressive episode(s) is not better explained by schizoaffective disorder, schizophrenia, schizophreniform disorder, delusional disorder, or other specified or unspecified schizophrenia spectrum and other psychotic disorder.

    ii. The episode is not due to the physiological effects of a substance or another medical condition. However, a manic episode that both emerges during antidepressant treatment *and* persists beyond the physiological effect of the treatment meets criteria for bipolar I disorder.

c. Modifiers

    i. Current (or most recent) episode

- Manic [F31.x, 126–127]
- Hypomanic [F31.x, 126–127]
- Depressed [F31.x, 126–127]
- Unspecified [F31.9, 126–127]: Use when the symptoms, but not the duration, of an episode meet criteria.

    ii. Specifiers

- With anxious distress
- With mixed features: At least three of the symptoms of a major depressive episode are present simultaneously.
- With rapid cycling
- With melancholic features
- With atypical features
- With mood-congruent psychotic features
- With mood-incongruent psychotic features
- With catatonia
- With peripartum onset
- With seasonal pattern

    iii. Course and severity

- Current or most recent episode manic, hypomanic, depressed, unspecified
- Mild, moderate, severe

- With psychotic features
- In partial remission, in full remission
- Unspecified

d. Alternatives

   i. If a substance, including a substance prescribed to treat depression, directly causes the episode, consider substance/medication-induced bipolar and related disorder [F1x.xx, 142–145].

   ii. If another medical condition causes the episode, consider bipolar and related disorder due to another medical condition [F06.3x, 145–147].

2. Bipolar II Disorder [F31.81, 132–139]

   For a diagnosis of bipolar II disorder, it is necessary to meet criteria for at least one hypomanic episode. The hypomanic episode may have been preceded by and may be followed by major depressive episodes.

   a. Inclusion: A hypomanic episode—defined as a distinct period of abnormally and persistently elevated or irritable mood and increased goal-directed activity or energy, lasting at least 4 days and present most of the day—requires the presence of at least <u>three</u> of the following symptoms.

      i. Inflated self-esteem or grandiosity: *During that period, did you feel especially confident, as though you could accomplish something extraordinary that you could not have done otherwise?*

      ii. Decreased need for sleep: *During that period, did you notice any change in how much sleep you needed to feel rested? Did you feel rested after less than 3 hours of sleep?*

      iii. More talkative than usual: *During that period, did anyone tell you that you talked more than usual or that it was hard to interrupt you?*

      iv. Flight of ideas: *During that period, were your thoughts racing? Did you have so many ideas that you could not keep up with them?*

      v. Distractibility: *During that period, were you having more trouble than usual focusing? Did you find yourself easily distracted?*

      vi. Increased goal-directed activity: *During that period, how did you spend your time? Did you find yourself much more active than usual?*

vii. Excessive involvement in activities that have a high potential for painful consequences: *During that period, did you engage in activities that were unusual for you? Did you spend money, use substances, or engage in sexual activities in a way that is unusual for you? Did any of these activities cause trouble for anyone?*

b. Exclusions

i. If there has ever been a manic episode or if the episode is attributable to the physiological effects of a substance/medication, do not use this diagnosis.

ii. If the hypomanic episode is better explained by schizoaffective disorder, schizophrenia, schizophreniform disorder, delusional disorder, or other specified or unspecified schizophrenia spectrum and other psychotic disorder, do not use this diagnosis.

iii. If the hypomanic episode is severe enough to cause marked impairment in social or occupational functioning or to necessitate hospitalization, do not use this diagnosis.

c. Modifiers

i. Specify current or most recent episode

- Hypomanic
- Depressed

ii. Specifiers

- With anxious distress
- With mixed features: At least three of the symptoms of a major depressive episode are present simultaneously.
- With rapid cycling
- With mood-congruent psychotic features
- With mood-incongruent psychotic features
- With catatonia
- With peripartum onset
- With seasonal pattern

iii. Course

- In partial remission
- In full remission

iv. Severity

- Mild

- Moderate
- Severe

d. Alternatives

  i. If a person reports 1 or more years of multiple hypomanic and depressive symptoms that never rose to the level of a hypomanic or major depressive episode, consider cyclothymic disorder [F34.0, 139–141]. During the same 1-year period, the hypomanic and depressive periods have been present for at least half the time, and the individual has not been without the symptoms for more than 2 months at a time. If the symptoms are due to the physiological effects of a substance or another medical condition, do not use this diagnosis.

  ii. If a person experiences symptoms characteristic of bipolar disorder that cause clinically significant distress or functional impairment without meeting full criteria for a bipolar disorder, consider unspecified bipolar and related disorder [F31.9, 149]. If you wish to communicate the specific reason a person's symptoms do not meet the criteria, as in short-duration hypomania, short-duration cyclothymia, and hypomania without prior major depressive episode, consider other specified bipolar and related disorder [F31.89, 148].

Depressive Disorders

DSM-5 pp. 155–188

Screening question: *Have you been feeling sad, blue, down, depressed, or irritable? If so: Does feeling this way make it hard to do things, hard to concentrate, or difficult to sleep?*

If yes, ask: *Did those times ever last at least 2 weeks? Did these periods ever cause you significant trouble with your friends or family, at work, or in another setting?*

- If yes, proceed to major depressive disorder criteria.

1. Major Depressive Disorder [F3x.xx, 160–168]

   a. Inclusion: Requires the presence of at least <u>five</u> of the following symptoms, which must include either depressed mood or loss of interest or pleasure (anhedo-nia), during the same 2-week episode.

  i. Depressed mood most of the day (already assessed)
 ii. Markedly diminished interest in activities or plea-sures (already assessed)
iii. Significant weight loss or gain: *During that period, did you notice any change in your appetite? Did you notice any change in your weight?*
 iv. Insomnia or hypersomnia: *During that period, how much and how well were you sleeping?*
  v. Psychomotor agitation or retardation: *During that period, did anyone tell you that you seemed to move faster or slower than usual?*
 vi. Fatigue or loss of energy: *During that period, what was your energy level like? Did anyone tell you that you seemed worn down or less energetic than usual?*
vii. Feelings of worthlessness or excessive guilt: *During that period, did you feel tremendous regret or guilt about current or past events or relationships?*
viii. Diminished concentration: *During that period, were you able to make decisions or concentrate like you usu-ally do?*
 ix. Recurrent thoughts of death or suicide: *During that period, did you think about death more than you usually do? Have you thought about hurting yourself or taking your own life?*

b. Exclusions

  i. If the person has ever had a manic episode or a hy-pomanic episode, or the major depressive episode is attributable to the physiological effects of a sub-stance or to another medical condition, do not use this diagnosis.
 ii. If the major depressive episode is better explained by schizoaffective disorder, schizophrenia, schizo-phreniform disorder, delusional disorder, or other specified or unspecified schizophrenia spectrum and other psychotic disorder, do not use this diag-nosis.

c. Modifiers

  i. Specifiers

    • With anxious distress

- With mixed features: At least three of the symptoms of a major depressive episode are present simultaneously.
- With melancholic features
- With atypical features
- With mood-congruent psychotic features
- With mood-incongruent psychotic features
- With catatonia
- With peripartum onset
- With seasonal pattern

ii. Course and severity

- Single episode
- Recurrent episode
- Mild [F3x.0, 162]
- Moderate [F3x.1, 162]
- Severe [F3x.2, 162]
- With psychotic features [F3x.3, 162]
- In partial remission [F3x.4x, 162]
- In full remission [F3x.xx, 162]
- Unspecified [F3x.9, 162]

d. Alternatives

i. If a person reports experiencing depression or anhedonia for at least 1 year, resulting in clinically significant distress or impairment, along with at least two of the symptoms of a major depressive episode, consider persistent depressive disorder (dysthymia) [F34.1, 168–171]. If a person experiences 2 continuous months without depressive symptoms, do not use this diagnosis. If the person has ever had symptoms that met the criteria for a bipolar disorder or a cyclothymic disorder, do not use this diagnosis. If the disturbance is better explained by a psychotic disorder or is due to the physiological effects of a substance or another medical condition, do not use this diagnosis.

ii. If the episode is directly caused by a substance, including a substance prescribed to treat depression, consider a substance/medication-induced depressive disorder [F1x.x4, 175–180].

iii. If another medical condition causes the episode, consider a depressive disorder due to another medical condition [F06.3x, 180–183].

iv. If a person experiences a depressive episode that causes clinically significant distress or functional impairment without meeting full criteria for a depressive disorder, consider unspecified depressive disorder [F32.9, 184]. To communicate the specific reason a person's symptoms do not meet the criteria, consider other specified depressive disorder [F32.8, 183–184]. Examples include recurrent brief depression and depressive episode with insufficient symptoms.

Anxiety Disorders

DSM-5 pp. 189–233

Screening questions: *During the past several months, have you frequently been worried about a number of things in your life? Is it hard for you to control or stop your worrying? Have you ever felt suddenly frightened, nervous, or anxious for no reason at all?*

If yes, ask: *Are there specific things, places, or social situations that make you feel very anxious or tearful?*

- If a specific phobia is elicited, proceed to specific phobia disorder criteria.
- If not, first proceed to panic disorder criteria. Then proceed to generalized anxiety disorder criteria.

1. Specific Phobia [F40.2xx, 197–202]

    a. Inclusion: Requires that for at least 6 months, a person has experienced marked fear or anxiety characterized by the following <u>three</u> symptoms.

    i. Specific fear: *Do you fear a specific object or situation such as flying, heights, animals, or something else so much that being exposed to it makes you feel immediately afraid or anxious? What is it?*

    ii. Fear or anxiety provoked by exposure: *When you encounter [this object or situation], do you cry or experience an immediate sense of fear or anxiety?*

    iii. Avoidance: *Do you find yourself taking steps to avoid [this object or situation]? What are they? When you have to encounter [this object or situation], do you experience intense fear or anxiety?*

b. Exclusion: The fear, anxiety, and avoidance are not restricted to objects or situations related to obsessions, reminders of traumatic events, separation from home or attachment figures, or social situations.

c. Modifiers

    i. Specifiers

- Animal
- Natural environment
- Blood-injection injury
- Situational
- Other

d. Alternatives

    i. If an older person reports developmentally inappropriate and excessive distress when separated from home or a major attachment figure, or expresses persistent worry that such a figure will be harmed or die, resulting in reluctance or refusal to be separated from home or the major attachment figure, consider separation anxiety disorder [F93.0, 190–195]. The minimum duration of symptoms necessary to meet the diagnostic criteria is 6 months for adults.

    ii. If a person reports at least 6 months of marked and disproportionate fear or anxiety about situations such as public transportation, open spaces, being in shops or theaters, standing in line or being in a crowd, or being outside the home alone, and if these fears cause her to actively avoid these situations, consider agoraphobia [F40.00, 217–221].

    iii. If a person reports at least 6 months of marked fear or anxiety about, or avoidance of, social situations in which she fears that other people will observe or scrutinize her out of proportion to the actual threat posed by these situations, these social situations provoke fear or anxiety, and these situations are either avoided or endured, consider social anxiety disorder (social phobia) [F40.10, 202–208].

2. Panic Disorder [F41.0, 208–214]

a. Inclusion: Requires recurrent panic attacks, as characterized by at least <u>four</u> of the following symptoms.

i. Palpitations, pounding heart, or accelerated heart rate: *When you experience these sudden surges of intense fear or discomfort, does your heart race or pound?*

ii. Sweating: *During these events, do you find yourself sweating more than usual?*

iii. Trembling or shaking: *During these events, do you shake or develop a tremor?*

iv. Sensations of shortness of breath or smothering: *During these events, do you feel as though you are being smothered or cannot catch your breath?*

v. Feelings of choking: *During these events, do you feel as though you are choking, as if something is blocking your throat?*

vi. Chest pain or discomfort: *During these events, do you feel intense pain or discomfort in your chest?*

vii. Nausea or abdominal distress: *During these events, do you feel sick to your stomach or as if you need to vomit?*

viii. Feeling dizzy, unsteady, light-headed, or faint: *During these events, do you feel dizzy, light-headed, or as if you may faint?*

ix. Chills or heat sensations: *During these events, do you feel very cold and shiver, or do you feel intensely hot?*

x. Paresthesias: *During these events, do you feel numbness or tingling?*

xi. Derealization or depersonalization: *During these events, do you feel as if people or places that are familiar to you are unreal or that you are so detached from your body that it is as if you are standing outside your body or watching yourself?*

xii. Fear of losing control or "going crazy": *During these events, do you fear you may be losing control, or even "going crazy"?*

xiii. Fear of dying: *During these events, do you fear you may be dying?*

b. Inclusion: At least one panic attack is followed by at least 1 month of at least <u>one</u> of the following symptoms.

i. Persistent concern or worry about additional panic attacks or their consequences: *Are you persistently concerned or worried about additional panic attacks? Are you persistently concerned or worried that these attacks mean you are having a heart attack, losing control, or "going crazy?"*

    ii. Maladaptive behavior change to avoid attacks: *Have you made significant changes in your behavior, such as avoiding unfamiliar situations or exercise, in order to avoid attacks?*

  c. Exclusion: If the disturbance is better explained by another mental disorder or is attributable to the physiological effects of a substance/medication or another medical condition, do not use this diagnosis.

  d. Alternative: If a person reports panic attacks as described above but neither experiences persistent worry about consequences nor makes maladaptive changes to avoid attacks, consider using the panic attack specifier (DSM-5, pp. 214–217). This specifier can be used with other anxiety disorders, as well as with depressive, traumatic, and substance use disorders.

3. Generalized Anxiety Disorder [F41.1, 222–226]

  a. Inclusion: Requires excessive anxiety and worry that is difficult to control, occurring more days than not for at least 6 months, about a number of events or activities (e.g., work performance), associated with at least <u>three</u> of the following symptoms.

    i. Restlessness: *When you think about events or activities that make you anxious or worried, do you feel restless, on edge, or "keyed up?"*

    ii. Being easily fatigued: *Do you find that you often tire or fatigue easily?*

    iii. Difficulty concentrating: *When you are anxious or worried, do you often find it hard to concentrate or find that your mind goes blank?*

    iv. Irritability: *When you are anxious or worried, do you often feel irritable or easily annoyed?*

    v. Muscle tension: *When you get anxious or worried, do you often experience muscle tightness or tension?*

    vi. Sleep disturbance: *Do you find it difficult to fall asleep or stay asleep, or do you experience restless and unsatisfying sleep?*

  b. Exclusion: If the anxiety and worry are better explained by another mental disorder or are attributable to the physiological effects of a substance/medication or another medical condition, do not use this diagnosis.

c. Alternatives

    i. If the episode is directly caused by a substance, including a medication prescribed to treat a mental disorder, consider a substance/medication-induced anxiety disorder [F1x.x8x, 226–230].

    ii. If another medical condition directly causes the anxiety and worry, consider an anxiety disorder due to another medical condition [F06.4, 230–232].

    iii. If a person experiences symptoms characteristic of an anxiety disorder that cause clinically significant distress or functional impairment without meeting full criteria for another anxiety disorder, consider unspecified anxiety disorder [F41.9, 233]. If you wish to communicate the specific reason a person's symptoms do not meet the criteria for a specific anxiety disorder, consider other specified anxiety disorder [F41.8, 233]. Examples include generalized anxiety not occurring more days than not and *ataque de nervios* (attack of nerves).

Obsessive-Compulsive and Related Disorders

DSM-5 pp. 235–264

Screening questions: *Do you ever get unwanted thoughts, urges, or pictures stuck in your mind that repeat, and you cannot make them stop? Is there anything you feel you have to check, clean, or organize over and over again in order to feel OK?*

If yes, ask: *Do these experiences or behaviors ever cause you significant trouble with your friends or family, at work, or in another setting?*

- If yes, proceed to obsessive-compulsive disorder criteria.
- If no, proceed to the body-focused repetitive behavior screening question, which follows the obsessive-compulsive disorder section below.

1. Obsessive-Compulsive Disorder [F42, 237–242]

    a. Inclusion: Requires the presence of obsessive thoughts, compulsive behaviors, or both, as manifested by the following symptoms.

i. Obsessive thoughts: *When you experience these un-wanted images, thoughts, or urges, do they make you anxious or distressed? Do you have to work hard to ignore or suppress these kinds of thoughts?*

ii. Compulsive behaviors: *Some people try to reverse intrusive ideas by repeatedly performing some kind of action such as hand washing or lock checking, or by a mental act such as counting, praying, or silently repeating words. Do you do something like that? Do you think that doing so will reduce your distress or prevent something from occurring?*

b. Inclusion: The obsessions or compulsions are time-consuming (e.g., take more than 1 hour per day) or cause clinically significant distress or impairment.

c. Exclusions

i. If the obsessions or compulsions are better explained by another mental disorder, do not use this diagnosis.

ii. If the obsessive-compulsive symptoms are attributable to the direct physiological effects of a substance, do not use this diagnosis.

iii. If a person reports that her intrusive images, thoughts, or urges are pleasurable, she does not meet the criteria for an obsessive-compulsive disorder.

d. Modifiers

i. Specifiers

• Insight

— With good or fair insight: Use if a person recognizes that her obsessive-compulsive beliefs are definitely or probably untrue.

— With poor insight: Use if a person thinks her obsessive-compulsive beliefs are probably true.

— With absent insight/delusional beliefs: Use if a person is completely convinced that her obsessive-compulsive beliefs are true.

ii. Tic-related: Use if a person meets criteria for either a current or lifetime chronic tic disorder.

e. Alternatives

i. If a person reports intrusive images, thoughts, or urges centered on her body image, consider body dysmorphic disorder [F45.22, 242–247]. The criteria include preoccupation with perceived defects in physical appearance beyond concern about weight or body fat in a person with an eating disorder, repetitive behaviors or mental acts in response to concern about appearance, and clinically significant distress or impairments because of the preoccupation.

ii.   If a person reports persistent difficulty in parting with possessions regardless of their value, consider hoarding disorder [F42, 247–251]. The criteria include strong urges to save items, distress associated with discarding items, and the accumulation of a large number of possessions that clutter the home or workplace to the extent that it can no longer be used for its intended function.

iii. If a substance, including a substance prescribed to treat depression, directly causes the condition, consider substance/medication-induced obsessive-compulsive and related disorder [F1x.x88, 257–260].

iv.   If another medical condition directly causes the episode, consider obsessive-compulsive and related disorder due to another medical condition [F06.8, 260–263].

v.   If a person reports intrusive images, thoughts, or urges centered on more real-world concerns, consider an anxiety disorder.

vi.   If a person experiences symptoms characteristic of an obsessive-compulsive and related disorder that cause clinically significant distress or functional impairment without meeting full criteria for another obsessive-compulsive and related disorder, consider unspecified obsessive-compulsive and related disorder [F42, 264]. If you wish to communicate the specific reason a person's symptoms do not meet the criteria for a specific obsessive-compulsive and related disorder, consider other specified obsessive-compulsive and related disorder [F42, 263–264]. Examples include body-focused repetitive behavior disorder, obsessional jealousy, and *koro* (anxiety that the penis or vulva and nipples will recede into the body).

2. Body-Focused Repetitive Behaviors

   a. Inclusion: DSM-5 includes two conditions, trichotillo-mania (hair-pulling disorder) [F63.3, 251–254] and ex-coriation (skin-picking) disorder [L98.1, 254–257], with identically structured criteria. Either diagnosis requires the presence of <u>all three</u> of the following symptoms, plus distress or impairment caused by the symptoms.

      i. Behavior: *Do you frequently pull your hair or pick at your skin so much that it has caused hair loss or skin lesions?*

      ii. Repeated attempts to change: *Have you repeatedly tried to decrease or stop this behavior?*

      iii. Impairment: *Does this behavior cause you to feel ashamed or out of control? Do you avoid social settings because of this behavior?*

   b. Alternative: If the behavior is associated with another medical condition or mental disorder or is the result of substance use, the behavior should be diagnosti-cally accounted for with those conditions and you should not diagnose either trichotillomania or excori-ation disorder.

Trauma- and Stressor-Related Disorders

DSM-5 pp. 265–290

Screening questions: *What is the worst thing that has ever happened to you? Has someone ever touched you in a way you did not want? Have you ever felt that your life was in danger or thought that you were going to be seriously injured? Do you have unhappy memories that make it hard to sleep or to feel OK now?*

If yes, ask: *Do you think about or relive these events? Does thinking about these experiences ever cause significant trouble with your friends or family, at work, or in another setting?*

• If yes, proceed to posttraumatic stress disorder criteria.

1. Posttraumatic Stress Disorder [F43.10, 271–280]

   a. Inclusion: Requires exposure to actual or threatened death, serious injury, or sexual violation. The exposure can be firsthand or witnessed. The exposure can also be from learning about violent or accidental trauma experienced by a close friend or family member. Finally, the exposure can be repeated or extreme exposure to aversive details of a traumatic event. In addition, a person must experience at least <u>one</u> of the following intrusion symptoms for at least 1 month after the traumatic experience.

   i. Memories: *After that experience, did you ever experience intrusive memories when you did not want to think about it?*

   ii. Dreams: *Did you have recurrent, distressing dreams related to the experience?*

  iii. Flashbacks: *After that experience, did you ever feel as if it were happening to you again, as in a flashback?*

  iv. Exposure distress: *When you are around people, places, or objects that remind you of that experience, do you feel intense or prolonged distress?*

   v. Physiological reactions: *When you are around people, places, or objects that remind you of that experience, do you have distressing physical responses?*

b. Inclusion: In addition, a person must experience at least <u>one</u> of the following avoidance symptoms after the traumatic experience.

   i. Internal reminders: *Do you work hard to avoid thoughts, feelings, or physical sensations that bring up memories of this experience?*

   ii. External reminders: *Do you work hard to avoid people, places, and objects that bring up memories of this experience?*

c. Inclusion: In addition, a person must experience at least <u>two</u> of the following negative symptoms.

   i. Impaired memory: *Do you have trouble remembering important parts of the experience?*

   ii. Negative self-image: *Do you frequently think negative thoughts about yourself, other people, or the world?*

  iii. Blame: *Do you frequently blame yourself or others for your experience, even when you know that you or they were not responsible?*

  iv. Negative emotional state: *Do you stay down, angry, ashamed, or fearful most of the time?*

     v. Decreased participation: *Are you much less inter-ested in activities in which you used to participate?*

    vi. Detachment: *Do you feel detached or estranged from people in your life because of this experience?*

  vii. Inability to experience positive emotion: *Do you find that you cannot feel happy, loved, or satisfied? Do you feel numb, or that you cannot love?*

d. Inclusion: In addition, a person must experience at least <u>two</u> of the following arousal behaviors.

     i. Irritability or aggressiveness: *Do you often act very grumpy or become aggressive?*

    ii. Recklessness: *Do you often act reckless or self-destructive?*

   iii. Hypervigilance: *Are you always on edge or keyed up?*

   iv. Exaggerated startle: *Do you startle easily?*

    v. Impaired concentration: *Do you often have trouble concentrating on a task or problem?*

   vi. Sleep disturbance: *Do you often have difficulty fall-ing asleep or staying asleep, or do you often wake up without feeling rested?*

e. Exclusion: If the episode is directly caused by the use of a substance or by another medical condition, do not use this diagnosis.

f. Modifiers

     i. Subtypes

       • With dissociative symptoms: depersonalization
       • With dissociative symptoms: derealization

    ii. Specifier

       • With delayed expression: Person does not exhibit all the diagnostic criteria until at least 6 months after the traumatic experience.

g. Alternatives

     i. If the episode lasts less than 1 month and the ex-perience occurred within the past month, and the person experiences at least <u>nine</u> of the posttrau-matic symptoms enumerated above, consider acute stress disorder [F43.0, 280–286].

    ii. If the episode began within 3 months of the expe-rience and a person does not meet the symptom-atic and behavioral criteria for posttraumatic stress disorder, consider an adjustment disorder

[F43.2x, 286–289]. The criteria include marked distress disproportionate to an acute stressor, either traumatic or nontraumatic, and significant impairment in function.

iii. If a person experiences symptoms characteristic of a trauma- and stressor-related disorder that cause clinically significant distress or functional impairment without meeting full criteria for one of the named disorders, consider unspecified trauma- and stressor-related disorder [F43.9, 290]. If you wish to communicate the specific reason a person's symptoms do not meet the criteria for a specific disorder, consider other specified trauma- and stressor-related disorder [F43.8, 289]. Examples include adjustment-like disorder with delayed onset of symptoms that occur more than 3 months after the stressor.

Dissociative Disorders

DSM-5 pp. 291–307

Screening questions: *Everyone has trouble remembering things sometimes, but do you ever lose time, forget important details about yourself, or find evidence that you took part in events that you cannot recall? Do you ever feel as if people or places that are familiar to you are unreal? Do you ever feel as if you are standing outside your body or watching yourself? Do you lose track of time and feel unsure of what you did during that time?*

If yes, ask: *Did these experiences ever cause you significant trouble with your friends or family, at work, or in another setting?*

• If amnesia predominates, proceed to dissociative amnesia criteria.
• If depersonalization or derealization predominates, proceed to depersonalization/derealization disorder criteria.

1. Dissociative Amnesia [F44.0, 298–302]

   a. Inclusion: Requires the presence of inability to recall important autobiographical information beyond ordinary forgetting, most often manifested by at least <u>one</u> of the following symptoms.

      i. Localized or selective amnesia: *Do you find yourself unable to recall a really important event, especially an event that was very stressful or even traumatic?*

      ii. Generalized amnesia: *Do you find yourself unable to recall really important moments in your life history or details of your very identity?*

  b. Exclusions

      i. If the disturbance is better accounted for by a major or mild neurocognitive disorder, dissociative identity disorder, posttraumatic stress disorder, acute stress disorder, or somatic symptom disorder, do not use this diagnosis.

      ii. If the disturbance is due to the physiological effects of a substance or a neurological or other medical condition, do not use this diagnosis.

  c. Modifiers

      i. Specifier

        • With dissociative fugue [F44.1, 298]: Person engages in purposeful travel or bewildered wandering for which she has amnesia.

  d. Alternative: If a person reports a disruption of identity, characterized by two or more distinct personality states or an experience of possession that causes clinically significant distress and functional impairment, consider dissociative identity disorder [F44.81, 292–298]. The criteria include recurrent gaps in recall that are inconsistent with ordinary forgetting and dissociative experiences that are not a normal part of a broadly accepted cultural or religious practice and that are not attributable to the physiological effects of a substance or another medical condition.

2. Depersonalization/Derealization Disorder [F48.1, 302–306]

  a. Inclusion: Requires at least <u>one</u> of the following manifestations.

      i. Depersonalization: *Do you frequently have experiences of unreality or detachment—as if you are an outside observer of your mind, thoughts, feelings, sensations, body, or whole self?*

      ii. Derealization: *Do you frequently have experiences of unreality or detachment from your surroundings? For*

example, do you often experience people or places as un-
real, dreamlike, foggy, lifeless, or visually distorted?

b. Inclusion: Requires intact reality testing. *During these experiences, can you distinguish the experiences from actual events—what is occurring outside of you?*

c. Exclusions

  i. If the disturbance is due to the physiological effects of a substance or a neurological or other medical condition, do not use this diagnosis.

  ii. If depersonalization or derealization occurs exclusively as symptoms of or during the course of another mental disorder, do not use this diagnosis.

d. Alternatives: If a person is experiencing a disorder whose most prominent symptoms are amnestic but does not meet the criteria for a specific disorder, consider unspecified dissociative disorder [F44.9, 307]. If you wish to communicate the specific reason a person's symptoms do not meet criteria for a specific disorder, consider other specified dissociative disorder [F44.89, 306–307]. Examples include chronic and recurrent syndromes of mixed dissociative symptoms, identity disturbances in individuals subjected to prolonged periods of intense coercive persuasion, acute reactions to stressful situations, and dissociative trance.

Somatic Symptom and Related Disorders

DSM-5 pp. 309–327

Screening questions: *Do you worry about your health more than most people? Do you get sick with aches and pains more often than most people your age?*

If yes, ask: *Do these experiences significantly affect your daily life?*

If yes, ask: *Which is worse for you, worrying about the symptoms you experience or worrying about your health and the possibility that you are sick?*

• If worry about symptoms predominates, proceed to somatic symptom disorder criteria.

- If worry about being ill or sick predominates, proceed to illness anxiety disorder criteria.

1. Somatic Symptom Disorder [F45.1, 311–315]

   a. Inclusion: Requires at least <u>one</u> somatic symptom that is distressing. *Do you experience symptoms that cause you to feel anxious or distressed? Do these symptoms significantly disrupt your daily life?*

   b. Inclusion: Requires at least <u>one</u> of the following thoughts, feelings, or behaviors, for at least 6 months.

      i. Disproportionate thoughts: *How serious are your health concerns, and do you think about them often?*

      ii. Persistently high level of anxiety: *Do you persistently feel a high level of anxiety or worry about your health concerns?*

      iii. Excessive investment: *Do you find yourself investing a lot more time and energy into your health concerns than you would like to do?*

   c. Modifiers

      i. Specifiers

         - With predominant pain
         - Persistent

      ii. Severity

         - Mild: One of the additional symptoms specified in inclusion criterion b above
         - Moderate: Two or more of the additional symptoms specified in inclusion criterion b above
         - Severe: Two or more of the additional symptoms specified in inclusion criterion b above plus multiple somatic complaints (or one very severe somatic symptom)

   d. Alternatives

      i. If a person is focused on the loss of bodily function rather than on the distress a particular symptom causes, consider conversion disorder (functional neurological symptom disorder) [F44.x, 318–321]. The criteria for this disorder include symptoms or deficits affecting voluntary motor or sensory function, clinical evidence that these symptoms or deficits are inconsistent with a recognized medical or neurological disease, and significant impairment in social or occupational functioning.

ii. If a person has a documented medical condition but behavioral or psychological factors adversely affect the course of her medical condition by delaying recovery, decreasing adherence, significantly increasing health risks, or influencing the underlying pathophysiology, consider psychological factors affecting other medical conditions [F54, 322–324].

iii. If a person falsifies physical or psychological signs or symptoms or induces injury or disease to deceptively present herself to others as ill, impaired, or injured, consider factitious disorder imposed on self [F68.10, 324–326]. If a person exhibits these behaviors in pursuit of obvious external rewards, as in malingering, do not use this diagnosis. If a person's symptoms are better accounted for by another mental disorder, do not use this diagnosis.

iv. If a person falsifies physical or psychological signs or symptoms or induces injury or disease to deceptively present someone else to others as ill, impaired, or injured, consider factitious disorder imposed on another [F68.10, 324–326]. This diagnosis is assigned to the perpetrator rather than the victim. If the perpetrator exhibits these behaviors in pursuit of obvious external rewards, as in malingering, do not use this diagnosis. If the perpetrator's behavior is better accounted for by another mental disorder, do not use this diagnosis.

2. Illness Anxiety Disorder [F45.21, 315–318]

a. Inclusion: Requires <u>all</u> of the following symptoms for at least 6 months and the <u>absence</u> of somatic symptoms.

i. Preoccupation: *Do you find yourself unable to stop thinking about having or acquiring a serious illness?*

ii. Anxiety: *Do you feel a high level of anxiety or worry about having or acquiring a serious illness?*

iii. Associated behaviors: *How have these worries affected your behavior? Some people find themselves frequently checking their body for signs of illness; reading about illness all the time; or avoiding persons, places, or objects to ward off illness. Are you doing any of those things or other similar things?*

b. Exclusion: If a person's symptoms are better explained by another mental disorder, do not use this diagnosis.

c. Modifiers

i. Subtypes
   • Care-seeking type
   • Care-avoidant type

d. Alternatives: If a person endorses symptoms characteristic of a somatic symptom and related disorder that cause clinically significant distress or impairment without meeting the full criteria for a specific disorder, consider unspecified somatic symptom and related disorder [F45.9, 327]. If you wish to communicate the specific reason a person's symptoms do not meet criteria for a specific disorder, consider other specified somatic symptom and related disorder [F45.8, 327]. Examples include brief somatic symptom disorder, brief illness anxiety disorder, and illness anxiety disorder without excessive health-related behaviors.

Feeding and Eating Disorders

DSM-5 pp. 329–354

Screening questions: *What do you think of your appearance? Do you ever restrict or avoid particular foods so much that your health or weight is negatively affected?*
If yes, ask: *When you consider yourself, is the shape or weight of your body one of the most important things about you?*

• If yes, proceed to anorexia nervosa criteria.
• If no, proceed to avoidant/restrictive food intake disorder criteria.

1. Anorexia Nervosa [F50.0x, 338–345]

a. Inclusion: Requires the presence of <u>all three</u> of the following features.

i. Energy restriction leading to significantly low body weight adjusted for age, developmental trajectory, physical health, and sex: *Have you limited* the food you eat to achieve a low body weight? What was the least you ever weighed? What do you weigh now?

ii. Fear of weight gain or behavior interfering with weight gain: *Do you have an intense fear of gaining weight or becoming fat? Has there ever been a time when you were already at a low weight and still did things to interfere with gaining weight?*

iii. Disturbance in self-perceived weight or shape: *How do you experience the weight and shape of your body? How do you think having a significantly low body weight will affect your physical health?*

b. Modifiers

 i. Subtypes

 • Restricting type [F50.01, 339]: Use when a person reports no recurrent episodes of binge eating or purging in the last 3 months.
 • Binge-eating/purging type [F50.02, 339]: Use when a person reports recurrent episodes of binge eating or purging in the last 3 months.

 ii. Specifiers

 • In partial remission
 • In full remission

 iii. Severity

 • Mild: Body mass index (BMI) $\geq$17 kg/m^2
 • Moderate: BMI 16–16.99 kg/m^2
 • Severe: BMI 15–15.99 kg/m^2
 • Extreme: BMI <15 kg/m^2

c. Alternative: If a person reports recurrent binge eating, recurrent inappropriate compensatory behaviors to prevent weight gain (e.g., misuse of laxatives or other medications, self-induced vomiting, excessive exercise), and self-image unduly influenced by body shape or weight, consider bulimia nervosa [F50.2, 345–350]. The diagnosis requires that binge eating and compensatory behaviors both occur, on average, at least once a week for 3 months. If binge eating and compensating behaviors occur only during episodes of anorexia nervosa, do not use this diagnosis.

2. Avoidant/Restrictive Food Intake Disorder [F50.8, 334–338]

a. Inclusion: Requires significant disturbance in eating or feeding manifested by persistent failure to meet appropriate nutritional and/or energy needs associated with at least <u>one</u> of the following sequelae.

    i. Significant weight loss: *Do you avoid certain foods or restrict what you eat to the extent that you have experienced a significant weight loss?*

    ii. Significant nutritional deficiency: *Do you avoid or restrict food to the extent that doing so has negatively affected your health, as in causing a significant nutritional deficiency?*

    iii. Dependence on enteral feeding or oral supplements: *Have you avoided or restricted food to the extent that you depend on tube feedings or oral supplements to maintain nutrition?*

    iv. Marked interference with psychosocial functioning: *Can you eat with other people or participate in social activities when food is present? Has avoiding or restricting food impaired your ability to participate in your usual social activities or made it hard to form or sustain relationships?*

b. Exclusions

    i. If the eating disturbance is better explained by lack of available food, by an associated culturally sanctioned practice, or by eating practices related to a disturbance in body image, do not use this diagnosis.

    ii. If the eating disturbance is due to another medical condition or is better explained by another mental condition, do not use this diagnosis.

c. Alternatives

    i. If a person persistently eats nonfood substances over a period of at least 1 month, consider pica [F50.8, 329–331]. If the eating of nonnutritive, nonfood substances is part of a culturally supported or socially normative practice, do not use this diagnosis.

    ii. If a person repeatedly regurgitates food over a period of at least 1 month, consider rumination disorder [F98.21, 332–333]. If the regurgitation occurs as the result of an associated gastrointestinal or other medical condition or occurs exclusively during the course of anorexia nervosa, bulimia nervosa, binge-eating disorder, or avoidant/restrictive food intake disorder, do not use this diagnosis.

iii. If a person has an atypical, mixed, or subthreshold disturbance in eating and feeding or if you lack sufficient information to make a more specific diagnosis, consider unspecified feeding or eating disorder [F50.9, 354]. DSM-5 also allows the use of this category for specific syndromes that are not formally included. If you wish to communicate the specific reason a person's symptoms do not meet criteria for a specific disorder, consider other specified feeding or eating disorder [F50.8, 353–354]. Examples include atypical anorexia nervosa, binge-eating disorder, and purging disorder.

Sleep-Wake Disorders

DSM-5 pp. 361–422

Screening questions: *Is your sleep often inadequate or of poor quality? Alternatively, do you often experience excessive sleepiness? Have you, or someone else, noticed any unusual behaviors while you sleep? Have you, or someone else, noticed that you stop breathing or gasp for air while sleeping?*

- If dissatisfaction with sleep quantity or quality predominates, proceed to insomnia disorder criteria.
- If excessive sleep predominates, proceed to hypersomnolence disorder criteria.
- If an irrepressible need to sleep or sudden lapses into sleep predominate, proceed to narcolepsy criteria.
- If sleep-breathing problems predominate, proceed to obstructive sleep apnea hypopnea criteria.
- If unusual sleep behaviors (parasomnias) predominate, proceed to restless legs syndrome criteria.

1. Insomnia Disorder [G47.00, 362–368]

   a. Inclusion: Requires dissatisfaction with sleep quantity or quality, at least 3 nights per week, for at least 3 months, as manifested by at least <u>one</u> of the following symptoms.

      i. Difficulty initiating sleep: *Do you often have trouble getting to sleep?*

    ii. Difficulty maintaining sleep: *Once asleep, do you frequently awaken when you do not want to? Do you have trouble returning to sleep after these awakenings?*

    iii. Early-morning awakening: *Do you often wake up earlier than you intended and find yourself unable to return to sleep?*

b. Exclusions

    i. If a person does not have adequate opportunity for sleep, do not use this diagnosis.

    ii. If the physiological effects of a substance cause a person's insomnia, do not use this diagnosis.

    iii. If a person's insomnia is better explained by another sleep-wake disorder, another mental disorder, or another medical condition, do not use this diagnosis.

c. Modifiers

    i. Specifiers

- With non–sleep disorder mental comorbidity, including substance use disorders
- With other medical comorbidity
- With another sleep disorder

    ii. Course

- Episodic: Symptoms last 1–3 months
- Persistent: Symptoms last 3 months or longer
- Recurrent: At least two episodes within 1 year

d. Alternatives

    i. If a person experiences a persistent or recurrent pattern of sleep disruption leading to excessive sleepiness, insomnia, or both and this disruption is due primarily to an alteration of the circadian system or to a misalignment between the endogenous circadian rhythm and the sleep-wake schedule required by a person's physical environment or her social or professional schedule, consider a circadian rhythm sleep-wake disorder [G47.2x, 390–398]. The sleep disturbance must cause clinically significant distress or functional impairment. Subtypes include delayed sleep phase type, advanced sleep phase type, and irregular sleep-wake type.

ii. If substance use, intoxication, or withdrawal is etiologically related to insomnia that causes significant distress or impairment, consider substance/
medication-induced sleep disorder, insomnia type
[F1x.x82, 413–420]. If the insomnia is better accounted for by delirium, a non–substance-induced
sleep disorder, or the sleep symptoms usually associated with an intoxication or withdrawal syndrome, do not use this diagnosis.

iii. If a person experiences symptoms characteristic of
an insomnia disorder that cause clinically significant distress or impairment without meeting criteria for a disorder, consider unspecified insomnia
disorder [G47.00, 420–421]. If you wish to communicate specific reasons that full criteria are not met,
consider other specified insomnia disorder [G47.09,
420]. Examples include brief insomnia disorder and
insomnia restricted to nonrestorative sleep.

2. Hypersomnolence Disorder [G47.10, 368–372]

a. Inclusion: Requires excessive sleepiness at least three
times per week for at least 3 months, despite a main sleep
period lasting at least 7 hours, that causes significant distress or functional impairment. The hypersomnolence is
manifested by at least <u>one</u> of the following symptoms.

i. Recurrent periods of sleep: *Do you often have several periods of sleep within the same day?*

ii. Prolonged nonrestorative sleep episode: *When you
sleep for at least 9 hours, do you still wake up without
feeling refreshed or restored?*

iii. Sleep inertia: *Do you often have difficulty being fully
awake? After awakening, do you often feel groggy or
notice that you have trouble engaging in tasks or activities that would otherwise be simple for you?*

b. Exclusion: If the hypersomnia occurs exclusively during the course of another sleep disorder, is better accounted for by another sleep disorder, or is
attributable to the physiological effects of a substance,
do not use this diagnosis.

c. Modifiers

i. Specifiers

• With mental disorder (including substance use
disorders)

- With medical condition
- With another sleep disorder

ii. Course

- Acute: Duration of less than 1 month
- Subacute: Duration of 1–3 months
- Persistent: Duration of more than 3 months

iii. Severity

- Mild: Difficulty maintaining daytime alertness 1–2 days/week
- Moderate: Difficulty maintaining daytime alertness 3–4 days/week
- Severe: Difficulty maintaining daytime alertness 5–7 days/week

d. Alternative: If substance use, intoxication, or withdrawal is etiologically related to daytime sleepiness, consider substance/medication-induced sleep disorder, daytime sleepiness type [F1x.x82, 413–420]. If the disturbance is better accounted for by delirium, a non–substance-induced sleep disorder, or sleep symptoms usually associated with an intoxication or withdrawal syndrome, do not use this diagnosis.

3. Narcolepsy [G47.4xx, 372–378]

a. Inclusion: Requires periods of an irrepressible need to sleep or lapsing into sleep, at least three times per week over the past 3 months, along with at least <u>one</u> of the following.

i. Episodes of cataplexy: *At least a few times a month, do you find that all of a sudden you grimace, open your mouth wide and thrust out your tongue, or lose muscle tone throughout your body?*

ii. Hypocretin deficiency: Measured using cerebrospinal fluid (CSF) hypocretin-1 immunoreactivity values.

iii. Nocturnal sleep polysomnography showing rapid eye movement (REM) sleep latency of 15 minutes or less or a multiple sleep latency test showing mean sleep latency of 8 minutes or less and two or more sleep-onset REM periods.

b. Modifiers

  i. Specifiers

   • Narcolepsy without cataplexy but with hypo-cretin deficiency: Low CSF hypocretin-1 levels and positive polysomnography/multiple sleep latency test result, but no cataplexy

   • Narcolepsy with cataplexy but without hypo-cretin deficiency: Cataplexy and positive poly-somnography/multiple sleep latency test result but normal CSF hypocretin-1 levels

   • Autosomal dominant cerebellar ataxia, deafness, and narcolepsy: Subtype caused by exon 21 DNA (cytosine-5)-methyltransferase-1 muta-tions and characterized by late-onset (age 30–40 years) narcolepsy (with low or intermediate CSF hypocretin-1 levels), deafness, cerebellar ataxia, and eventually dementia

   • Autosomal dominant narcolepsy, obesity, and type 2 diabetes: Narcolepsy, obesity, and type 2 diabetes and low CSF hypocretin-1 levels asso-ciated with a mutation in the myelin oligoden-drocyte glycoprotein gene

   • Narcolepsy secondary to another medical con-dition: Narcolepsy developing secondary to medical conditions that cause infectious (e.g., Whipple's disease, sarcoidosis), traumatic, or tumoral destruction of hypocretin neurons

  ii. Severity

   • Mild: Infrequent cataplexy (less than once per week), need for naps only once or twice per day, and less disturbed nocturnal sleep

   • Moderate: Cataplexy once daily or every few days, disturbed nocturnal sleep, and need for multiple naps daily

   • Severe: Drug-resistant cataplexy with multiple attacks daily, nearly constant sleepiness, and disturbed nocturnal sleep (i.e., movements, in-somnia, and vivid dreaming)

4. Obstructive Sleep Apnea Hypopnea [G47.33, 378–383]

 a. Inclusion: Requires repeated episodes of upper air-way obstruction during sleep. There must be polysomnographic evidence of at least five obstructive apneas or hypopneas per hour of sleep and <u>either</u> of the following symptoms.

  i. Nocturnal breathing disturbances: *Do you often disturb your partner or anyone else with snoring, snorting, gasping for air, or breathing pauses during sleep?*

  ii. Daytime sleepiness, fatigue, or nonrestorative sleep that is not attributable to another medical condition or is not explained by psychiatric morbidity: *When you have sufficient opportunity to get sleep, do you still wake up feeling exhausted, sleepy, or fatigued?*

b. Inclusion: Alternatively, the diagnosis can be made by polysomnographic evidence of 15 or more obstructive apneas or hypopneas per hour of sleep regardless of accompanying symptoms.

c. Modifiers

  i. Severity

   • Mild: Apnea hypopnea index value <15
   • Moderate: Apnea hypopnea index value of 15–30
   • Severe: Apnea hypopnea index value >30

d. Alternatives

  i. If a person has five or more central apneas per hour of sleep during polysomnographic examination and this disturbance is not better accounted for by another current sleep disorder, consider central sleep apnea [G47.31, 383–386].

  ii. If a person has episodes of shallow breathing associated with arterial oxygen desaturation and/or elevated carbon dioxide levels during polysomnographic examination and this disturbance is not better accounted for by another current sleep disorder, consider sleep-related hypoventilation [G47.3x, 387–390]. This disorder is most commonly associated with medical or neurological disorders, obesity, medication use, or substance use disorders.

5. Restless Legs Syndrome [G25.81, 410–413]

a. Inclusion: Requires an urge to move the legs, usually accompanied by or in response to uncomfortable and unpleasant sensations in the legs, at least three times per week for at least 3 months, as manifested by <u>all</u> of the following symptoms.

    i. Urge to move legs: *While you are asleep, do you often experience uncomfortable or unpleasant sensations in the legs? Do you often experience an urge to move your legs when you are otherwise inactive?*

    ii. Relieved with movement: *Are these symptoms partially or completely relieved by moving your legs?*

    iii. Nocturnal worsening: *What times of day do you most experience the urge to move your legs? Is it worse in the evening or at night, no matter what you have done during the day?*

b. Exclusions

    i. If a person's restless legs are better explained by another mental disorder, another medical condition, or a behavioral condition, do not use this diagnosis.

    ii. If the physiological effects of a substance cause restless legs, do not use this diagnosis.

c. Alternatives

    i. If a person experiences recurrent episodes of incomplete awakening from sleep in which she has an abrupt and terrifying awakening (sleep terror) or she rises from bed and walks about (sleepwalking), usually during the first third of the major sleep episode, consider non–rapid eye movement sleep arousal disorder [F51.x, 399–404]. When experiencing an episode, the person experiences little to no dream imagery. The person experiences amnesia for the episode and is relatively unresponsive to efforts of other people.

    ii. If a person repeatedly experiences extremely dysphoric and well-remembered dreams and rapidly becomes alert and oriented on awakening from these dysphoric dreams, consider nightmare disorder [F51.5, 404–407]. The dream disturbance or the sleep disturbance produced by awakening from the nightmare causes clinically significant distress or functional impairment. If the dysphoric dreams occur exclusively during another mental disorder or as the physiological effect of a substance or another medical condition, do not use this diagnosis.

iii. If a person repeatedly experiences episodes of arousal from sleep associated with vocalization and/or complex motor behaviors sufficient to result in injury to herself or her bed partner, consider rapid eye movement sleep behavior disorder [G47.52, 407–410]. These behaviors arise during REM sleep and typically occur more than 90 minutes after sleep onset. On awakening, the person is fully awake, alert, and oriented. The diagnosis requires either polysomnographic evidence of REM sleep disturbance or a history suggestive of REM sleep behavior disorder in the context of an established synucleinopathy diagnosis.

iv. If substance use, intoxication, or withdrawal is etiologically related to daytime sleepiness, consider substance/medication-induced sleep disorder, parasomnia type [F1x.x82, 413–420]. If the disturbance is better accounted for by delirium, a non–substance-induced sleep disorder, or the sleep symptoms usually associated with an intoxication or withdrawal syndrome, do not use this diagnosis.

v. If a person experiences symptoms characteristic of restless legs syndrome or another parasomnia that causes clinically significant distress or impairment without meeting criteria for a disorder, consider unspecified insomnia disorder [G47.00, 420–421]. If you wish to communicate specific reasons that full criteria are not met, consider other specified insomnia disorder [G47.09, 420].

Sexual Dysfunctions

DSM-5 pp. 423–450

Screening question: *Have you been less interested in sex than usual or experienced difficulties in sexual performance?*

If yes, ask: *Have these experiences lasted at least 6 months and caused you significant distress or impairment?*

- If disinterest in sex predominates, proceed to female sexual interest/arousal disorder criteria for women or male hypoactive sexual desire disorder for men.

- If difficulties in sexual performance predominate, proceed to female orgasmic disorder for women or erectile disorder for men.

1. Erectile Disorder [F52.21, 426–429)

   a. Inclusion: Requires the presence of at least <u>one</u> of the following symptoms on almost all or all occasions of sexual activity, for at least 6 months.

      i. Difficulty obtaining erection: *During sexual activity, have you noticed a marked difficulty in obtaining an erection?*

      ii. Difficulty maintaining erection: *Do you have a marked difficulty in maintaining an erection until the completion of sexual activity?*

      iii. Decrease in erectile rigidity that interferes with activity: *Have you experienced a decrease in the rigidity of your erections severe enough that it interferes with sexual activity?*

   b. Exclusion: If a man has sexual dysfunction that is better accounted for by a nonsexual mental disorder, severe relationship distress, or another significant stressor or is attributable to the effects of a substance/medication or another medical condition, do not use this diagnosis.

   c. Modifiers

      i. Subtypes

         - Generalized: Not limited to certain types of stimulation, situations, or partners
         - Situational: Occurs only with certain types of stimulation, situations, or partners

      ii. Specifiers

         - Lifelong: Disturbance has been present since the individual became sexually active.
         - Acquired: Disturbance began after a period of relatively normal sexual function.

      iii. Severity

         - Mild: Evidence of mild distress over the symptoms
         - Moderate: Evidence of moderate distress over the symptoms
         - Severe: Evidence of severe or extreme distress over the symptoms

d. Alternatives

    i. If a man reports that during almost all or all partnered sexual experiences over at least the last 6 months, he either did not ejaculate or experienced a marked delay in ejaculation, consider delayed ejaculation [F52.32, 424–426]. If the symptoms are better explained by a nonsexual mental disorder or severe relationship distress, do not use this diagnosis.

    ii. If a man reports that he ejaculated within approximately 1 minute following vaginal penetration during almost all or all partnered experiences over at least the last 6 months, without wishing to do so, consider premature (early) ejaculation [F52.4, 443–446].

2. Female Orgasmic Disorder [F52.31, 429–432]

a. Inclusion: Requires the presence of <u>one</u> of the following symptoms during all or almost all sexual experiences, for at least 6 months.

    i. Delayed, absent, or infrequent orgasms: *Does it take you much longer than usual to achieve orgasm, or do you rarely or never experience an orgasm?*

    ii. Reduced intensity of orgasms: *Have you noticed the intensity of your orgasms is markedly reduced?*

b. Exclusion: If a woman has sexual dysfunction that is better explained by a nonsexual mental disorder, severe relationship distress, or another significant stressor or is attributable to the effects of a substance/medication or another medical condition, do not use this diagnosis.

c. Modifiers

    i. Subtypes

- Generalized: Not limited to certain types of stimulation, situations, or partners
- Situational: Occurs only with certain types of stimulation, situations, or partners

    ii. Specifiers

- Lifelong: Disturbance has been present since the individual became sexually active.
- Acquired: Disturbance began after a period of relatively normal sexual function.
- Never experienced an orgasm in any situation.

iii. Severity

   - Mild: Evidence of mild distress over the symptoms
   - Moderate: Evidence of moderate distress over the symptoms
   - Severe: Evidence of severe or extreme distress over the symptoms

d. Alternative: If a woman reports at least 6 months of marked difficulty having vaginal intercourse; marked vulvovaginal or pelvic pain during vaginal intercourse; marked fear or anxiety about vulvovaginal or pelvic pain in anticipation of, during, or as a result of vaginal penetration; or marked tensing or tightening of the pelvic floor muscles during attempted vaginal penetration, consider genito-pelvic pain/penetration disorder [F52.6, 437–440].

3. Female Sexual Interest/Arousal Disorder [F52.22, 433–437]

   a. Inclusion: Requires at least 6 months with absent or reduced sexual interest or arousal as manifested by at least <u>three</u> of the following symptoms.

      i. Absent/reduced sexual interest: *Have you noticed that the intensity or frequency of your interest in sexual activity is absent or markedly reduced?*

      ii. Absent/reduced sexual thoughts: *Have you noticed that the intensity or frequency of your sexual thoughts or fantasies is absent or markedly reduced?*

      iii. No/reduced sexual initiation: *Have you noticed that the intensity or frequency with which you initiate sexual activity or respond to a partner's initiation is absent or markedly reduced?*

      iv. Absent/reduced sexual excitement/pleasure: *When you engage in sexual encounters, have you noticed that almost all of the time, your experience of sexual excitement or pleasure is absent or markedly reduced?*

      v. Absent/reduced sexual response: *Have you noticed that the intensity or frequency with which you experience sexual interest in response to erotic signals is absent or markedly reduced?*

      vi. Absent/reduced sexual sensations: *When you engage in sexual encounters, have you noticed that almost all of the time, the intensity or frequency with which you experience genital or nongenital sensations is absent or markedly reduced?*

b. Exclusion: If a woman has sexual dysfunction that is better accounted for by a nonsexual mental disorder, severe relationship distress, or another significant stressor or is attributable to the effects of a substance/medication or another medical condition, do not use this diagnosis.

c. Modifiers

   i. Subtypes
      - Generalized: Not limited to certain types of stimulation, situations, or partners
      - Situational: Occurs only with certain types of stimulation, situations, or partners

   ii. Specifiers
      - Lifelong: Disturbance has been present since the individual became sexually active.
      - Acquired: Disturbance began after a period of relatively normal sexual function.

   iii. Severity
      - Mild: Evidence of mild distress over the symptoms
      - Moderate: Evidence of moderate distress over the symptoms
      - Severe: Evidence of severe distress over the symptoms

d. Alternatives

   i. If a woman has a clinically significant disturbance in sexual function directly associated with the use or discontinuation of a substance or medication, consider a substance/medication-induced sexual dysfunction [F1x.x81, 446–450].

   ii. If a woman has a sexual dysfunction but the symptoms do not meet the threshold for another sexual dysfunction diagnosis, the etiology is uncertain, or there is insufficient information to diagnose a current sexual dysfunction, consider unspecified sexual dysfunction [F52.9, 450]. If you wish to communicate the specific reason a woman's symptoms do not meet full criteria, consider other specified sexual dysfunction [F52.8, 450].

4. Male Hypoactive Sexual Desire Disorder [F52.0, 440–443]

   a. Inclusion: Requires persistently or recurrently defi-cient (or absent) sexual thoughts or fantasies and de-sire for sexual activity for at least 6 months. *Have you noticed that the intensity or frequency of your sexual thoughts, desires, or fantasies is absent or markedly re-duced?*

   b. Exclusion: If a man has sexual dysfunction that is bet-ter accounted for by a nonsexual mental disorder, se-vere relationship distress, or another significant stressor or is attributable to the effects of a substance/ medication or another medical condition, do not use this diagnosis.

   c. Modifiers

      i. Subtypes

         • Generalized: Not limited to certain types of stimulation, situations, or partners
         • Situational: Occurs only with certain types of stimulation, situations, or partners

      ii. Specifiers

         • Lifelong: Disturbance has been present since the individual became sexually active.
         • Acquired: Disturbance began after a period of relatively normal sexual function.

      iii. Severity

         • Mild: Evidence of mild distress over the symp-toms
         • Moderate: Evidence of moderate distress over the symptoms
         • Severe: Evidence of severe or extreme distress over the symptoms

   d. Alternatives

      i. If a man has a clinically significant disturbance in sexual function directly associated with the use or discontinuation of a substance or medication, con-sider a substance/medication-induced sexual dysfunction [F1x.x81, 446–450).

      ii. If a man has a sexual dysfunction but the symp-toms do not meet the threshold for another sexual dysfunction diagnosis, the etiology is uncertain, or there is insufficient information to diagnose a current sexual dysfunction, consider unspecified sexual dysfunction [F52.9, 450]. If you wish to communicate the specific reason the symptoms do not meet full criteria, consider other specified sexual dysfunction [F52.8, 450].

Gender Dysphoria

DSM-5 pp. 451–459

Screening question: *Are you really uncomfortable with your assigned gender?*

If yes, ask: *Has this discomfort lasted at least 6 months and gotten to the point where you really feel that your given gender is incongruent with your gender identity? Does this discomfort cause significant trouble with your friends or family, at work, or in another setting?*

1. Gender Dysphoria in Adults [F64.1, 452–459]

   a. Inclusion: Requires at least <u>two</u> of the following manifestations for at least 6 months.

      i. Incongruence: *Have you experienced a profound sense that your primary or secondary sex characteristics do not match your gender identity?*

      ii. Desire to change: *Have you experienced a profound desire to change your primary or secondary sex characteristics because they do not match your gender identity?*

      iii. Desire to have sex characteristics of other gender: *Have you experienced a strong desire to have the primary or secondary sex characteristics that match your experience of gender?*

      iv. Desire to be another gender: *Have you experienced a strong desire to be of a gender other than your given gender?*

      v. Desire to be treated as another gender: *Have you experienced a strong desire to be treated as a gender other than your given gender?*

      vi. Conviction that one has feelings of another gender: *Have you experienced a strong conviction that your typical feelings and reactions are those of a gender other than your given gender?*

b. Modifiers

   i. Specifiers

      • With a disorder of sex development.
      • Posttransition: The individual has transitioned to full-time living in the desired gender (with or without legalization of gender change) and has undergone (or is preparing to have) at least one cross-sex medical procedure or treatment regimen.

c. Alternatives: If a person experiences symptoms characteristic of gender dysphoria that cause clinically significant distress or impairment without meeting the full criteria for gender dysphoria, consider unspecified gender dysphoria [F64.9, 459]. If you wish to communicate the specific reason a person's symptoms do not meet full criteria, consider other specified gender dysphoria [F64.8, 459].

Disruptive, Impulse-Control, and Conduct Disorders

DSM-5 pp. 461–480

Screening questions: *Do you often become so upset that you make threats to hurt other people, animals, or property? Have you ever intentionally hurt people or animals, destroyed property, tricked other people, or stolen things?*

If yes, ask: *Have these behaviors ever caused you significant trouble with your friends or family, or work, with the authorities, or in another setting?*

• If recurrent behavioral outbursts predominate, proceed to intermittent explosive disorder criteria.

1. Intermittent Explosive Disorder [F63.81, 466–469]

   a. Inclusion: Requires recurrent behavioral outbursts in which a person does not control aggressive impulses as manifested by <u>either</u> of the following.

i. Verbal or physical aggression: *Over the past 3 months, have you had impulsive outbursts in which you were verbally or physically aggressive toward other people, animals, or property? Have these outbursts occurred, on average, at least twice weekly?*

ii. Three behavioral outbursts involving damage to or destruction of property and/or physical assault: *Over the past 12 months, have you had at least three impulsive outbursts where you lost control of your behavior and assaulted other people or destroyed property?*

b. Inclusion: Also requires <u>all</u> <u>three</u> of the following.

i. Magnitude of aggressiveness is disproportionate to any provocation or psychosocial stressor: *If you look back at these outbursts, can you identify any events or stressors that you associate with them? Was your response much more aggressive or extreme than these events or stressors?*

ii. Recurrent outbursts are neither premeditated nor in pursuit of a tangible objective: *When you had these outbursts, did they happen when you were feeling angry or impulsive? Did the outburst occur without a clear goal, such as obtaining money or intimidating someone?*

iii. Outbursts cause marked personal distress, impair occupational or interpersonal functioning, or are associated with financial or legal consequences: *How do these outbursts affect how you feel about yourself and how you get along with friends, family, and other people in your life? Have you ever suffered financial or legal consequences because of your outbursts?*

c. Exclusions

i. If the recurrent aggressive outbursts are fully explained by another mental disorder or are attributable to another medical condition or to the physiological effects of a substance/medication, do not use this diagnosis.

ii. If aggressive behavior occurs only in the context of an adjustment disorder, do not use this diagnosis.

d. Alternatives

i. If a person reports deliberate and purposeful fire setting on at least two occasions, consider pyromania [F63.1, 476–477]. The diagnosis requires tension or affective arousal before the fire setting, fascination with fire, and pleasure or relief when setting or witnessing fires. If the fire setting is done for monetary gain, to conceal criminal activity, out of anger, or in response to a hallucination, do not use this diagnosis. If the fire setting is better explained by intellectual disability, conduct disorder, mania, or antisocial personality disorder, do not use this diagnosis.

ii. If a person repeatedly fails to resist impulses to steal objects that are not needed for her personal use or their monetary value, consider kleptomania [F63.3, 478–479]. The diagnosis requires tension or affective arousal before the theft and pleasure or relief at the time of the theft. If the stealing is done out of anger or vengeance or in response to a hallucination, do not use this diagnosis. If the stealing is better explained by conduct disorder, mania, or antisocial personality disorder, do not use this diagnosis.

iii. If recurrent rule breaking predominates, consider conduct disorder [F91.x, 469–475]. Conduct disorder requires a repetitive and persistent pattern of behavior in which the basic rights of others or major age-appropriate societal norms or rules are violated. The onset of the disorder typically occurs in childhood or adolescence.

iv. If a person exhibits at least 6 months of a persistent pattern of angry and irritable mood along with defiant and vindictive behavior, consider oppositional defiant disorder [F91.3, 462–466]. The onset of the disorder typically occurs in childhood or adolescence.

v. If a person exhibits symptoms characteristic of a disruptive, impulse-control, and conduct disorder that cause clinically significant distress or impairment without meeting the full criteria for a diagnosis named above, consider unspecified disruptive, impulse-control, and conduct disorder [F91.9, 480]. If you wish to communicate the specific reason a person does not meet the full criteria, consider other specified disruptive, impulse-control, and conduct disorder [F91.8, 479].

Substance-Related and Addictive Disorders

Screening questions: *How often do you drink alcohol? On the average day when you have at least one drink, how many drinks do you have? Have you had any problems as a result of drinking? When you stop drinking, do you go through withdrawal?*

Repeat for illicit and prescription drugs; begin by asking: *Have you ever experimented with drugs?*

After asking about drugs, ask: *Do you bet, wager, or gamble in a way that interferes with your life?*

If yes, ask: *Did these experiences ever cause you significant trouble with your friends or family, at work, or in another setting?*

- If a person reports problems with substance use, proceed to the substance use disorder criteria for each particular substance.
- If a person presents with substance intoxication, proceed to the substance intoxication criteria for each particular substance.
- If a person reports problems with substance withdrawal, proceed to the substance withdrawal criteria for each particular substance.

1. Alcohol Use Disorder [F10.x0, 490–497]

    a. Inclusion: Requires a problematic pattern of alcohol use leading to clinically significant impairment or distress as manifested by at least <u>two</u> of the following symptoms in a 12-month period.

        i.   Drinking alcohol in larger amounts or over a longer period than intended: *When you drink, do you find that you drink more, and for a longer time, than you planned to?*

        ii. Persistent desire or unsuccessful effort to reduce alcohol use: *Do you want to cut back or stop drinking? Have you ever tried and failed to cut back or stop drinking alcohol?*

        iii. Great deal of time spent: *Do you spend a great deal of your time obtaining alcohol, drinking alcohol, or recovering from your alcohol use?*

iv. Cravings: *Do you experience strong cravings for or desires to drink alcohol?*

v. Failure to fulfill major role obligations: *Have you repeatedly failed to fulfill major obligations at work or home because of your alcohol use?*

vi. Continued use despite awareness of interpersonal or social problems: *Do you drink alcohol even though you suspect, or even know, that your use creates or worsens interpersonal or social problems?*

vii. Giving up activities for alcohol: *Are there important social, occupational, or recreational activities that you have given up or reduced because of your alcohol use?*

viii. Use in hazardous situations: *Have you repeatedly used alcohol in situations in which use could be physically hazardous, such as driving a car or operating a machine?*

ix. Continued use despite awareness of physical or psychological problems: *Do you drink alcohol even though you suspect, or even know, that your use creates or worsens problems with your mind and body?*

x. Tolerance as manifested by either of the following.

- Need for markedly increased amounts: *Do you find that in order to get intoxicated or achieve the desired effect of drinking, you need to consume much more alcohol than you used to?*
- Markedly diminished effects: *If you drink the same amount of alcohol as you used to, do you find that it has a lot less effect on you than it used to?*

xi. Withdrawal as manifested by either of the following.

- Characteristic alcohol withdrawal syndrome: *When you stop drinking, do you undergo withdrawal?*
- The same or a closely related substance is taken to relieve or avoid withdrawal symptoms: *Have you ever drunk alcohol or taken another substance to prevent alcohol withdrawal?*

b. Modifiers

i. Specifiers

- In early remission
- In sustained remission
- In a controlled environment

  ii. Severity

   • Mild [F10.10, 491]: Two to three symptoms are present
   • Moderate [F10.20, 491]: Four to five symptoms are present
   • Severe [F10.20, 491]: Six or more symptoms are present

 c. Alternative: If a person experiences problems associated with the use of alcohol that are not classifiable as alcohol use disorder, alcohol intoxication, alcohol withdrawal, alcohol intoxication delirium, alcohol withdrawal delirium, alcohol-induced neurocognitive disorder, alcohol-induced psychotic disorder, alcohol-induced bipolar disorder, alcohol-induced depressive disorder, alcohol-induced anxiety disorder, alcohol-induced sexual dysfunction, or alcohol-induced sleep disorder, consider unspecified alcohol-related disorder [F10.99, 503].

2. Alcohol Intoxication [F10.x29, 497–499]

 a. Inclusion: Requires at least <u>one</u> of the following signs or symptoms shortly after alcohol use.

   i. Slurred speech
   ii. Incoordination
   iii. Unsteady gait
   iv. Nystagmus
   v. Impairment in attention or memory
   vi. Stupor or coma

 b. Inclusion: Requires clinically significant problematic behavioral or psychological changes. *Since you began this episode of drinking, have you observed any significant changes in your behavior, mood, or judgment? Have you engaged in problematic activities or thought problematic thoughts that you would not have if you were sober?*

 c. Exclusion: If the symptoms are attributable to another medical condition or are better explained by another mental disorder, including intoxication with another substance, do not use this diagnosis.

3. Alcohol Withdrawal [F10.23x, 499–501]

 a. Inclusion: Requires at least <u>two</u> of the following symptoms developing within several hours to a few days of ceasing (or reducing) alcohol use that has been heavy and prolonged.

    i.   Autonomic hyperactivity

    ii. Increased hand tremor

    iii. Insomnia: *Over the past couple of days, have you found it more difficult than usual to get to sleep and to stay asleep?*

    iv. Nausea or vomiting: *Over the past couple of days, have you felt sick to your stomach, felt nauseated, or even vomited?*

    v. Transient visual, tactile, or auditory hallucinations or illusions: *Over the past couple of days, have you had any experiences where you worried that your mind was playing tricks on you, such as seeing, hearing, or feeling things that other people could not?*

    vi. Psychomotor agitation

    vii. Anxiety: *Over the past couple of days, have you felt more worried or anxious than usual?*

    viii. Generalized tonic-clonic seizures

b. Exclusion: If the symptoms are attributable to another medical condition or are better explained by another mental disorder, including intoxication with or withdrawal from another substance, do not use this diagnosis.

c. Modifiers

    i. Specifier

      • With perceptual disturbances [F10.232, 500]

4. Caffeine Intoxication [F15.929, 503–506]

a. Inclusion: Requires clinically significant problematic behavioral or psychological changes during, or shortly after, caffeine ingestion, usually in excess of 250 mg (e.g., 2–3 cups of brewed coffee), as manifested by at least <u>five</u> of the following signs or symptoms.

    i. Restlessness: *Over the past several hours, have you felt less able to remain at rest than usual?*

    ii. Nervousness: *Over the past several hours, have you felt more jittery or nervous than usual?*

    iii. Excitement: *Over the past several hours, have you felt more excited than usual?*

    iv. Insomnia: *Over the past several hours, if you tried to sleep, did you find it more difficult to get to sleep or stay asleep than usual?*

     v. Flushed face

    vi. Diuresis: *Over the past several hours, have you urinated more often or a greater amount than usual?*

   vii. Gastrointestinal disturbance: *Over the past several hours, have you experienced an upset stomach, nausea, vomiting, or diarrhea?*

  viii. Muscle twitching: *Over the past several hours, have you noticed your muscles twitching more than usual?*

    ix. Rambling flow of thought and speech: *Over the past several hours, have you or anyone else noticed that your thoughts or speech have been abnormally long-winded or even confused?*

     x. Tachycardia or cardiac arrhythmia

    xi. Periods of inexhaustibility: *Over the past several hours, have you felt as if you had so much energy that it could not be used up?*

   xii. Psychomotor agitation

b. Exclusion: If the symptoms are attributable to another medical condition or are better explained by another mental disorder, including intoxication with another substance, do not use this diagnosis.

c. Alternative: If a person experiences problems associated with the use of caffeine that are not classifiable as caffeine intoxication, caffeine withdrawal, caffeine-induced anxiety disorder, or caffeine-induced sleep disorder, consider unspecified caffeine-related disorder [F15.99, 509].

5. Caffeine Withdrawal [F15.93, 506–508]

a. Inclusion: Requires at least <u>three</u> of the following signs or symptoms developing within 24 hours of ceasing (or reducing) prolonged daily use of caffeine.

     i. Headache: *Over the past day, have you had any headaches?*

    ii. Marked fatigue or drowsiness: *Over the past day, have you felt extremely tired or sleepy?*

   iii. Dysphoric or depressed mood or irritability: *Over the past day, have you felt more down, depressed, or even more irritable than usual?*

   iv. Difficulty concentrating: *Over the past day, have you had difficulty staying focused on a task or activity?*

    v. Flu-like symptoms: *Over the past day, have you experienced flu-like symptoms, such as nausea, vomiting, or muscle pain or stiffness?*

b. Exclusion: If the symptoms are attributable to another medical condition or are better explained by another mental disorder, including intoxication with or withdrawal from another substance, do not use this diagnosis.

6. Cannabis Use Disorder [F12.x0, 509–516]

a. Inclusion: Requires a problematic pattern of cannabis use leading to clinically significant impairment or distress as manifested by at least <u>two</u> of the following in a 12-month period.

  i. Consuming cannabis in larger amounts or over a longer period than intended: *When you use cannabis, do you find that you use more, or for a longer time, than you planned to?*

  ii. Persistent desire or unsuccessful effort to reduce cannabis use: *Do you want to cut back or stop using cannabis? Have you ever tried and failed to cut back or stop using cannabis?*

  iii. Great deal of time spent: *Do you spend a great deal of your time obtaining cannabis, using cannabis, or recovering from your cannabis use?*

  iv. Cravings: *Do you experience strong desires or urges to use cannabis?*

  v. Failure to fulfill major role obligations: *Have you repeatedly failed to fulfill major obligations at work or home because of your cannabis use?*

  vi. Continued use despite awareness of interpersonal or social problems: *Do you use cannabis even though you suspect, or even know, that your use creates or worsens interpersonal or social problems?*

  vii. Giving up activities for cannabis: *Are there important social, occupational, or recreational activities that you have given up or reduced because of your cannabis use?*

  viii. Use in hazardous situations: *Have you repeatedly used cannabis in situations in which use could be physically hazardous, such as driving a car or operating a machine?*

  ix. Continued use despite awareness of physical or psychological problems: *Do you use cannabis even though you suspect, or even know, that your use creates or worsens problems with your mind and body?*

  x. Tolerance as manifested by <u>either</u> of the following.

- Markedly increased amounts: *Do you find that in order to get high or achieve the desired effect, you need to smoke or ingest much more cannabis than you used to?*
- Markedly diminished effects: *If you use the same amount of cannabis as you used to, do you find that it has a lot less effect on you than it used to?*

xi. Withdrawal as manifested by <u>either</u> of the following.

- Characteristic cannabis withdrawal syndrome: *When you stop using cannabis, do you undergo withdrawal?*
- The same or a closely related substance is taken to relieve or avoid withdrawal symptoms: *Have you used cannabis or another substance to prevent yourself from withdrawing from cannabis?*

b. Modifiers

i. Specifiers

- In early remission
- In sustained remission
- In a controlled environment

ii. Severity

- Mild [F12.10, 510]: Two or three symptoms are present.
- Moderate [F12.20, 510]: Four or five symptoms are present.
- Severe [F12.20, 510]: Six or more symptoms are present.

c. Alternative: If a person experiences problems associated with the use of cannabis that are not classifiable as cannabis use disorder, cannabis intoxication, cannabis withdrawal, cannabis intoxication delirium, cannabis withdrawal delirium, cannabis-induced neurocognitive disorder, cannabis-induced psychotic disorder, cannabis-induced bipolar disorder, cannabis-induced depressive disorder, cannabis-induced anxiety disorder, cannabis-induced sexual dysfunction, or cannabis-induced sleep disorder, consider unspecified cannabis-related disorder [F12.99, 519].

7. Cannabis Intoxication [F12.x2x, 516–517]

   a. Inclusion: Requires at least <u>two</u> of the following signs or symptoms shortly after cannabis use.

      i. Conjunctival injection
      ii. Increased appetite: *Over the past several hours, have you been much hungrier than usual?*
      iii. Dry mouth: *Over the past several hours, have you noticed that your mouth has been dry?*
      iv. Tachycardia

   b. Inclusion: Requires clinically significant problematic behavioral or psychological changes. *Since you began this episode of cannabis use, have you observed any significant changes in your mood, judgment, ability to interact with others, or sense of time? Have you engaged in problematic activities or thought problematic thoughts that you would not have without cannabis?*

   c. Exclusion: If the symptoms are attributable to another medical condition or are better explained by another mental disorder, including intoxication with another substance, do not use this diagnosis.

   d. Modifier

      i. With perceptual disturbances [F12.x22, 516]

8. Cannabis Withdrawal [F12.288, 517–519]

   a. Inclusion: Requires at least <u>three</u> of the following symptoms developing within 1 week of ceasing (or reducing) cannabis use that has been heavy and prolonged.

      i. Irritability, anger, or aggression: *Over the past week or so, have you felt more irritable or angry or that you were ready to confront or attack someone?*
      ii. Nervousness or anxiety: *Over the past week or so, have you felt more worried or anxious than usual?*
      iii. Sleep difficulty: *Over the past week or so, have you had any disturbing dreams or found it more difficult to get to sleep and to stay asleep than usual?*
      iv. Decreased appetite or weight loss: *Over the past week or so, have you been less hungry or even lost weight?*
      v. Restlessness: *Over the past week or so, have you felt less able to remain at rest than usual?*
      vi. Depressed mood: *Over the past week or so, have you felt more down or depressed than usual?*

vii. Somatic symptoms: *Over the past week or so, have you felt any unusual physical discomfort, such as stomach pain, tremors, sweating, fever, chills, or headaches?*

b. Exclusion: If the symptoms are attributable to another medical condition or are better explained by another mental disorder, including intoxication with or withdrawal from another substance, do not use this diagnosis.

9. Phencyclidine or Other Hallucinogen Use Disorder [F16.x0, 520–527]

a. Inclusion: Requires a problematic pattern of phencyclidine or other hallucinogen use leading to clinically significant impairment or distress as manifested by at least <u>two</u> of the following in a 12-month period.

i. Using phencyclidine or other hallucinogens in larger amounts or over a longer period than intended: *When you use hallucinogens, do you find that you use more, or for a longer time, than you planned to?*

ii. Persistent desire or unsuccessful effort to reduce hallucinogen use: *Do you want to cut back or stop using hallucinogens? Have you ever tried and failed to cut back or stop using hallucinogens?*

iii. Great deal of time spent: *Do you spend a great deal of your time obtaining hallucinogens, using hallucinogens, or recovering from your hallucinogen use?*

iv. Cravings: *Do you experience strong cravings for or desires to use hallucinogens?*

v. Failure to fulfill major role obligations: *Have you repeatedly failed to fulfill major obligations at work or home because of your hallucinogen use?*

vi. Continued use despite awareness of interpersonal or social problems: *Do you use hallucinogens even though you suspect, or even know, that your use creates or worsens interpersonal or social problems?*

vii. Giving up activities for hallucinogens: *Are there important social, occupational, or recreational activities that you have given up or reduced because of your hallucinogen use?*

viii. Use in hazardous situations: *Have you repeatedly used hallucinogens in situations in which use could be physically hazardous, such as driving a car or operating a machine?*

ix. Continued use despite awareness of physical or psychological problems: *Do you use hallucinogens even though you suspect, or even know, that your use creates or worsens problems with your mind and body?*

x. Tolerance as manifested by <u>either</u> of the following.

- Markedly increased amounts: *Do you find that in order to achieve the desired effect of hallucinogens, you need much more than you used to?*
- Markedly diminished effects: *If you use the same amount of a hallucinogen as you used to, do you find that it has a lot less effect on you than it used to?*

b. Modifiers

i. Specifiers

- In early remission
- In sustained remission
- In a controlled environment

ii. Severity (phencyclidine/other hallucinogen)

- Mild [F16.10, 521/524]: Two or three symptoms are present.
- Moderate [F16.20, 521/524]: Four or five symptoms are present.
- Severe [F16.20, 521/524]: Six or more symptoms are present.

c. Alternative: If a person experiences problems associated with the use of phencyclidine or another hallucinogen that are not classifiable as phencyclidine or other hallucinogen use disorder, phencyclidine or other hallucinogen intoxication, phencyclidine or other hallucinogen withdrawal, phencyclidine or other hallucinogen intoxication delirium, phencyclidine or other hallucinogen withdrawal delirium, phencyclidine or other hallucinogen-induced neurocognitive disorder, phencyclidine or other hallucinogen-induced psychotic disorder, phencyclidine or other hallucinogen-induced bipolar disorder, phencyclidine or other hallucinogen-induced depressive disorder, phencyclidine or other hallucinogen-induced anxiety disorder, phencyclidine or other hallucinogen-induced sexual dysfunction, or phencyclidine or other hallucinogen-induced sleep disorder, consider unspecified phencyclidine or other hallucinogen-related disorder [F16.99, 533].

10. Phencyclidine or Other Hallucinogen Intoxication [F16.x29, 527–530]

  a. Inclusion: Requires at least <u>two</u> of the following signs or symptoms shortly after phencyclidine or other hallucinogen use.

    Phencyclidine

    i. Vertical or horizontal nystagmus
    ii. Hypertension or tachycardia
    iii. Numbness or diminished responsiveness to pain
    iv. Ataxia
    v. Dysarthria
    vi. Muscle rigidity
    vii. Seizures or coma
    viii. Hyperacusis

    Other Hallucinogens

    i. Pupillary dilation
    ii. Tachycardia
    iii. Sweating: *Since taking the hallucinogen, have you noticed any change in how much you sweat?*
    iv. Palpitations: *Since taking the hallucinogen, has your heartbeat been more rapid, stronger, or more irregular than usual?*
    v. Blurring of vision: *Since taking the hallucinogen, has your vision been blurred?*
    vi. Tremors
    vii. Incoordination: *Since taking the hallucinogen, have you found it hard to coordinate your movements as you walk or otherwise move?*

  b. Inclusion: Requires clinically significant problematic behavioral or psychological changes. *Since you began this episode of hallucinogen use, have you observed any significant changes in your mood, judgment, ability to interact with others, or sense of time? Have you engaged in problematic activities or thought problematic thoughts that you would not have without hallucinogens?*

  c. Exclusion: If the symptoms are attributable to another medical condition or are better explained by another mental disorder, including intoxication with another substance, do not use this diagnosis.

11. Inhalant Use Disorder [F18.x0, 533–538]

   a. Inclusion: Requires a problematic pattern of inhalant use leading to clinically significant impairment or distress as manifested by at least <u>two</u> of the following in a 12-month period.

      i. Using inhalants in larger amounts or over a longer period than intended: *When you inhale, do you find that you use more inhalant, or for a longer time, than you planned to?*

      ii. Persistent desire or unsuccessful effort to reduce inhalant use: *Do you want to cut back or stop inhaling? Have you ever tried and failed to cut back or stop inhaling?*

      iii. Great deal of time spent: *Do you spend a great deal of your time obtaining inhalants, using inhalants, or recovering from your inhalant use?*

      iv. Cravings: *Do you experience strong cravings for or desires to use inhalants?*

      v. Failure to fulfill major role obligations: *Have you repeatedly failed to fulfill major obligations at work or home because of your inhalant use?*

      vi. Continued use despite awareness of interpersonal or social problems: *Do you use inhalants even though you suspect, or even know, that your use creates or worsens interpersonal or social problems?*

      vii. Giving up activities for inhalants: *Are there important social, occupational, or recreational activities that you have given up or reduced because of your inhalant use?*

      viii. Use in hazardous situations: *Have you repeatedly used inhalants in situations in which use could be physically hazardous, such as driving a car or operating a machine?*

      ix. Continued use despite awareness of physical or psychological problems: *Do you use inhalants even though you suspect, or even know, that your use creates or worsens problems with your mind and body?*

      x. Tolerance as manifested by <u>either</u> of the following.

         • Markedly increased amounts: *Do you find that in order to get high or achieve the desired effect of using inhalants, you need to use much more than you used to?*

- Markedly diminished effects: *If you inhale the same amount of an inhalant as you used to, do you find that it has a lot less effect on you than it used to?*

b. Modifiers

  i. Specifiers
    - In early remission
    - In sustained remission
    - In a controlled environment

  ii. Severity
    - Mild [F18.10, 534]: Two or three symptoms are present.
    - Moderate [F18.20, 534]: Four or five symptoms are present.
    - Severe [F18.20, 534]: Six or more symptoms are present.

c. Alternative: If a person experiences problems associated with the use of an inhalant that are not classifiable as inhalant use disorder, inhalant intoxication, inhalant withdrawal, inhalant intoxication delirium, inhalant withdrawal delirium, inhalant-induced neurocognitive disorder, inhalant-induced psychotic disorder, inhalant-induced bipolar disorder, inhalant-induced depressive disorder, inhalant-induced anxiety disorder, inhalant-induced sexual dysfunction, or inhalant-induced sleep disorder, consider unspecified inhalant-related disorder [F18.99, 540].

12. Inhalant Intoxication [F18.x29, 538–540]

a. Inclusion: Requires at least <u>two</u> of the following signs or symptoms after intended or unintended short-term, high-dose inhalant exposure.

  i. Dizziness: *Since using the inhalant, have you felt as if you were reeling or about to fall?*
  ii. Nystagmus
  iii. Incoordination: *Since using the inhalant, have you found it hard to coordinate your movements as you walk or otherwise move?*
  iv. Slurred speech
  v. Unsteady gait
  vi. Lethargy: *Since using the inhalant, have you felt very sleepy or had a marked lack of energy?*

vii. Depressed reflexes

viii. Psychomotor retardation

ix. Tremor

x. Generalized muscle weakness

xi. Blurred vision or diplopia: *Since using the inhalant, has your vision been blurred, or have you been seeing double?*

xii. Stupor or coma

xiii. Euphoria: *Since using the inhalant, have you felt mentally or physically elated or intensely excited or happy?*

b. Inclusion: Requires clinically significant problematic behavioral or psychological changes. *Since you began this episode of inhalant use, have you observed any significant changes in your mood, judgment, ability to interact with others, or sense of time? Have you engaged in problematic activities or thought problematic thoughts that you would not have without inhalants?*

c. Exclusion: If the symptoms are attributable to another medical condition or are better explained by another mental disorder, including intoxication with another substance, do not use this diagnosis.

13. Opioid Use Disorder [F11.x0, 541–546]

a. Inclusion: Requires a problematic pattern of opioid use leading to clinically significant impairment or distress as manifested by at least <u>two</u> of the following in a 12-month period.

i. Using opioids in larger amounts or over a longer period than intended: *When you use opioids, do you find that you use more, or for a longer time, than you planned to?*

ii. Persistent desire or unsuccessful effort to reduce opioid use: *Do you want to cut back or stop using opioids? Have you ever tried and failed to cut back or stop using opioids?*

iii. Great deal of time spent: *Do you spend a great deal of your time obtaining opioids, using opioids, or recovering from your opioid use?*

iv. Cravings: *Do you experience strong cravings for or desires to use opioids?*

v. Failure to fulfill major role obligations: *Have you repeatedly failed to fulfill major obligations at work or home because of your opioid use?*

    vi. Continued use despite awareness of interpersonal or social problems: *Do you continue to use opioids even though you suspect, or even know, that your use creates or worsens interpersonal or social problems?*

   vii. Giving up activities for opioid use: *Are there important social, occupational, or recreational activities that you have given up or reduced because of opioid use?*

  viii. Use in hazardous situations: *Have you repeatedly used opioids in situations in which use could be physically hazardous, such as driving a car or operating a machine?*

    ix. Continued use despite awareness of physical or psychological problems: *Do you use opioids even though you suspect, or even know, that your use creates or worsens problems with your mind and body?*

     x. Tolerance as manifested by <u>either</u> of the following.

- Markedly increased amounts: *Do you find that in order to get high or achieve the desired effect of using opioids, you need much more than you used to?*
- Markedly diminished effects (excluding opioid medications taken under medical supervision): *If you use the same amount of an opioid as you used to, do you find that it has a lot less effect on you than it used to?*

    xi. Withdrawal as manifested by <u>either</u> of the following.

- Characteristic opioid withdrawal syndrome: *When you stop using opioids, do you undergo withdrawal?*
- The same or a closely related substance is taken to relieve or avoid withdrawal symptoms: *Have you ever taken opioids or another substance to prevent opioid withdrawal?*

b. Modifiers

    i. Specifiers

- In early remission
- In sustained remission
- On maintenance therapy
- In a controlled environment

   ii. Severity

- Mild [F11.10, 542]: Two or three symptoms are present.

- Moderate [F11.20, 542]: Four or five symptoms are present.
- Severe [F11.20, 542]: Six or more symptoms are present.

c. Alternative: If a person experiences problems associated with the use of an opioid that are not classifiable as opioid use disorder, opioid intoxication, opioid withdrawal, opioid intoxication delirium, opioid withdrawal delirium, opioid-induced neurocognitive disorder, opioid-induced psychotic disorder, opioid-induced bipolar disorder, opioid-induced depressive disorder, opioid-induced anxiety disorder, opioid-induced sexual dysfunction, or opioid-induced sleep disorder, consider unspecified opioid-related disorder [F11.99, 550].

14. Opioid Intoxication [F11.x2x, 546–547]

a. Inclusion: Requires pupillary constriction shortly after opioid use and at least <u>one</u> of the following signs or symptoms.

   i. Drowsiness or coma
   ii. Slurred speech
   iii. Impairment in attention or memory

b. Inclusion: Requires clinically significant problematic behavioral or psychological changes. *Since you began this episode of opioid use, have you observed any significant changes in your mood, judgment, ability to interact with others, or sense of time? Have you engaged in problematic activities or thought problematic thoughts that you would not have without opioids?*

c. Exclusion: If the symptoms are attributable to another medical condition or are better explained by another mental disorder, including intoxication with another substance, do not use this diagnosis.

d. Modifier

   i. With perceptual disturbances [F11.x22, 546–547]

15. Opioid Withdrawal [F11.23, 547–549]

a. Inclusion: Requires at least <u>three</u> of the following symptoms developing within minutes to several days of ceasing (or reducing) opioid use that has been heavy and prolonged or following the administration of an opioid antagonist after a period of opioid use.

i. Dysphoric mood: *Over the past couple of days, have you been feeling more down or depressed than usual?*

ii. Nausea or vomiting: *Over the past couple of days, have you felt sick to your stomach, felt nauseated, or even vomited?*

iii. Muscle aches: *Over the past couple of days, have you experienced muscle aches or pains?*

iv. Lacrimation or rhinorrhea: *Over the past couple of days, have you noticed that you have been shedding tears when you did not feel like crying? Have you noticed that your nose has been running, or discharging clear fluid, more than usual?*

v. Pupillary dilation, piloerection, or sweating

vi. Diarrhea: *Over the past couple of days, have you experienced more frequent or more liquid stools than usual?*

vii. Yawning: *Over the past couple of days, have you been yawning much more than usual?*

viii. Fever

ix. Insomnia: *Over the past couple of days, have you found it more difficult than usual to get to sleep and to stay asleep?*

b. Exclusion: If the symptoms are attributable to another medical condition or are better explained by another mental disorder, including intoxication with or withdrawal from another substance, do not use this diagnosis.

16. Sedative, Hypnotic, or Anxiolytic Use Disorder [F13.x0, 550–556]

a. Inclusion: Requires a problematic pattern of sedative, hypnotic, or anxiolytic use leading to clinically significant impairment or distress as manifested by at least <u>two</u> of the following in a 12-month period.

i. Using sedatives, hypnotics, or anxiolytics in larger amounts or over a longer period than intended: *When you use sedatives, hypnotics, or anxiolytics, do you find that you use more, or for a longer time, than you planned to?*

ii. Persistent desire or unsuccessful effort to reduce sedative, hypnotic, or anxiolytic use: *Do you want to cut back or stop using sedatives, hypnotics, or anxiolytics? Have you ever tried and failed to cut back or stop use of these substances?*

iii. Great deal of time spent: *Do you spend a great deal of your time obtaining and using sedatives, hypnotics, or anxiolytics, or recovering from your sedative, hypnotic, or anxiolytic use?*

iv. Cravings: *Do you experience strong cravings for or desires to use sedatives, hypnotics, or anxiolytics?*

v. Failure to fulfill major role obligations: *Have you repeatedly failed to fulfill major obligations at work or home because of your sedative, hypnotic, or anxiolytic use?*

vi. Continued use despite awareness of interpersonal or social problems: *Do you use a sedative, hypnotic, or anxiolytic even though you suspect, or even know, that your use creates or worsens interpersonal or social problems?*

vii. Giving up activities for sedative, hypnotic, or anxiolytic use: *Are there important social, occupational, or recreational activities that you have given up or reduced because of your sedative, hypnotic, or anxiolytic use?*

viii. Use in hazardous situations: *Have you repeatedly used a sedative, hypnotic, or anxiolytic in situations in which use could be physically hazardous, such as driving a car or operating a machine?*

ix. Continued use despite awareness of physical or psychological problems: *Do you use sedatives, hypnotics, or anxiolytics even though you suspect, or even know, that your use creates or worsens problems with your mind and body?*

x. Tolerance as manifested by <u>either</u> of the following.

- Markedly increased amounts: *Do you find that in order to get intoxicated or achieve the desired effect of using sedatives, hypnotics, or anxiolytics, you need much more than you used to?*
- Markedly diminished effects: *If you use the same amount of a sedative, hypnotic, or anxiolytic as you used to, do you find that it has a lot less effect on you than it used to?*

xi. Withdrawal as manifested by <u>either</u> of the following.

- Characteristic sedative, hypnotic, or anxiolytic withdrawal syndrome: *When you stop using sedatives, hypnotics, or anxiolytics, do you undergo withdrawal?*
- The same or a closely related substance is taken to relieve or avoid withdrawal symptoms: *Have*

you ever taken sedatives, hypnotics, anxiolytics, or another substance to prevent withdrawal?

b. Modifiers

   i. Specifiers

   - In early remission
   - In sustained remission
   - In a controlled environment

   ii. Severity

   - Mild [F13.10, 552]: Two or three symptoms are present.
   - Moderate [F13.20, 552]: Four or five symptoms are present.
   - Severe [F13.20, 552]: Six or more symptoms are present.

c. Alternative: If a person experiences problems associated with the use of a sedative, hypnotic, or anxiolytic that are not classifiable as sedative, hypnotic, or anxiolytic use disorder; sedative, hypnotic, or anxiolytic intoxication; sedative, hypnotic, or anxiolytic withdrawal; sedative, hypnotic, or anxiolytic intoxication delirium; sedative, hypnotic, or anxiolytic withdrawal delirium; sedative-, hypnotic-, or anxiolytic-induced neurocognitive disorder; sedative-, hypnotic-, or anxiolytic-induced psychotic disorder; sedative-, hypnotic-, or anxiolytic-induced bipolar disorder; sedative-, hypnotic-, or anxiolytic-induced depressive disorder; sedative-, hypnotic-, or anxiolytic-induced anxiety disorder; sedative-, hypnotic-, or anxiolytic-induced sexual dysfunction; or sedative-, hypnotic-, or anxiolytic-induced sleep disorder, consider unspecified sedative-, hypnotic-, or anxiolytic-related disorder [F13.99, 560].

17. Sedative, Hypnotic, or Anxiolytic Intoxication [F13.x29, 556–557]

a. Inclusion: Requires <u>one</u> of the following signs or symptoms shortly after sedative, hypnotic, or anxiolytic use.

   i. Slurred speech
   ii. Incoordination
   iii. Unsteady gait
   iv. Nystagmus

     v. Impairment in cognition (i.e., attention or memory)
    vi. Stupor or coma

  b. Inclusion: Requires clinically significant maladaptive behavioral or psychological changes. *Since you began this episode of sedative, hypnotic, or anxiolytic use, have you observed any significant changes in your mood, judgment, ability to interact with others, or sense of time? Have you engaged in problematic activities or thought problematic thoughts that you would not have without sedatives, hypnotics, or anxiolytics?*

  c. Exclusion: If the symptoms are attributable to another medical condition or are better explained by another mental disorder, including intoxication with another substance, do not use this diagnosis.

18. Sedative, Hypnotic, or Anxiolytic Withdrawal [F13.23x, 557–560]

  a. Inclusion: Requires at least <u>two</u> of the following symptoms developing within several hours to a few days after ceasing (or reducing) sedative, hypnotic, or anxiolytic use that has been heavy and prolonged.

     i. Autonomic hyperactivity
    ii. Hand tremor
   iii. Insomnia: *Over the past couple of days, have you found it more difficult than usual to get to sleep and stay asleep?*
   iv. Nausea or vomiting: *Over the past couple of days, have you felt sick to your stomach, felt nauseated, or even vomited?*
    v. Transient visual, tactile, or auditory hallucinations or illusions: *Over the past couple of days, have you had any experiences where you worried that your mind was playing tricks on you, such as seeing, hearing, or feeling things that other people could not?*
   vi. Psychomotor agitation
  vii. Anxiety: *Over the past couple of days, have you felt more worried or anxious than usual?*
 viii. Grand mal seizures

  b. Exclusion: If the symptoms are attributable to another medical condition or are better explained by another mental disorder, including intoxication with or withdrawal from another substance, do not use this diagnosis.

    c. Modifier

       i. Specifier

         • With perceptual disturbances [F13.232, 558]

19. Stimulant Use Disorder [F1x.x0, 561–567]

    a. Inclusion: Requires a problematic pattern of stimulant use leading to clinically significant impairment or distress as manifested by at least <u>two</u> of the following in a 12-month period.

       i. Using stimulants in larger amounts or over a longer period than intended: *When you use stimulants, do you find that you use more, or for a longer time, than you planned to?*

       ii. Persistent desire or unsuccessful effort to reduce stimulant use: *Do you want to cut back or stop using stimulants? Have you ever tried and failed to cut back or stop using stimulants?*

       iii. Great deal of time spent: *Do you spend a great deal of your time obtaining stimulants, using stimulants, or recovering from your stimulant use?*

       iv. Cravings: *Do you experience strong cravings for or desires to use stimulants?*

       v. Failure to fulfill major role obligations: *Have you repeatedly failed to fulfill major obligations at home or work because of your stimulant use?*

       vi. Continued use despite awareness of interpersonal or social problems: *Do you use stimulants even though you suspect, or even know, that your use creates or worsens interpersonal or social problems?*

       vii. Giving up activities for stimulants: *Are there important social, occupational, or recreational activities that you have given up or reduced because of your stimulant use?*

       viii. Use in hazardous situations: *Have you repeatedly used stimulants in situations in which use could be physically hazardous, such as driving a car or operating a machine?*

       ix. Continued use despite awareness of physical or psychological problems: *Do you use stimulants even though you suspect, or even know, that your use creates or worsens problems with your mind and body?*

x. Tolerance as manifested by <u>either</u> of the following.
Note: This criterion is not met if patient is taking stimulants as prescribed under medical supervision.

- Markedly increased amounts: *Do you find that in order to get intoxicated or achieve the desired effect of using stimulants, you need much more than you used to?*
- Markedly diminished effects: *If you use the same amount of a stimulant as you used to, do you find that it has a lot less effect on you than it used to?*

xi. Withdrawal as manifested by <u>either</u> of the following.
Note: This criterion is not met if patient is taking stimulants as prescribed under medical supervision.

- Characteristic stimulant withdrawal syndrome: *When you stop using stimulants, do you undergo withdrawal?*
- The same or a closely related substance is taken to relieve or avoid withdrawal symptoms: *Have you ever taken stimulants or another substance to prevent withdrawal?*

b. Modifiers

i. Specify stimulant

- Amphetamine-type substance
- Cocaine
- Other or unspecified stimulant

ii. Specifiers

- In early remission
- In sustained remission
- In a controlled environment

iii. Severity

- Mild [F1x.10, 562]: Two or three symptoms are present.
- Moderate [F1x.20, 562]: Four or five symptoms are present.
- Severe [F1x.20, 562]: Six or more symptoms are present.

c. Alternative: If a person experiences problems associated with the use of a stimulant that are not classifiable as stimulant use disorder, stimulant intoxication, stimulant withdrawal, stimulant intoxication delirium, stimulant withdrawal delirium, stimulant-induced neurocognitive disorder, stimulant-induced psychotic disorder, stimulant-induced bipolar disorder, stimulant-induced depressive disorder, stimulant-induced anxiety disorder, stimulant-induced sexual dysfunction, or stimulant-induced sleep disorder, consider unspecified stimulant-related disorder [F1x.99, 570].

20. Stimulant Intoxication [F1x.x2x, 567–569]

   a. Inclusion: Requires at least <u>two</u> of the following signs or symptoms shortly after stimulant use.

      i. Tachycardia or bradycardia
      ii. Pupillary dilation
      iii. Elevated or lowered blood pressure
      iv. Perspiration or chills: *Over the past couple of hours, have you experienced chills or been sweating more than usual?*
      v. Nausea or vomiting: *Over the past couple of hours, have you felt sick to your stomach, felt nauseated, or even vomited?*
      vi. Evidence of weight loss
      vii. Psychomotor agitation
      viii. Muscular weakness, respiratory depression, chest pain, or cardiac arrhythmias
      ix. Confusion, seizures, dyskinesias, dystonias, or coma

   b. Inclusion: Requires clinically significant problematic behavioral or psychological changes. *Since you began this episode of stimulant use, have you observed any significant changes in your mood, judgment, ability to interact with others, or sense of time? Have you engaged in problematic activities or thought problematic thoughts that you would not have without stimulants?*

   c. Exclusion: If the symptoms are attributable to another medical condition or are better explained by another mental disorder, including intoxication with another substance, do not use this diagnosis.

   d. Modifiers

      i. Specifiers

         • Specify the intoxicant: amphetamine, cocaine, or other stimulant
         • With perceptual disturbances [F1x.x29, 567]

21. Stimulant Withdrawal [F1x.23, 569–570]

a. Inclusion: Requires the following symptom, developing within hours to days of ceasing (or reducing) stimulant use that has been heavy or prolonged.

   i. Dysphoric mood: *Over the past few hours or days, have you felt much more down or depressed than usual?*

b. Inclusion: Also requires at least <u>two</u> of the following symptoms developing simultaneously.

   i. Fatigue: *Over the past few hours or days, have you felt extremely sleepy or tired?*

   ii. Vivid, unpleasant dreams: *Over the past few hours or days, have you experienced unusually vivid, unpleasant dreams?*

   iii. Insomnia or hypersomnia: *Over the past few hours or days, have you found it more difficult than usual to get to sleep and stay asleep? Alternatively, have you found that you have been sleeping much more than usual?*

   iv. Increased appetite: *Over the past few hours or days, have you desired food much more than usual?*

   v. Psychomotor retardation or agitation

c. Exclusion: If the symptoms are attributable to another medical condition or are better explained by another mental disorder, including intoxication with or withdrawal from another substance, do not use this diagnosis.

d. Modifier

   i. Specifier

     • Specify the intoxicant: amphetamine, cocaine, or other stimulant

22. Tobacco Use Disorder [xxx.x, 571–574]

a. Inclusion: Requires a problematic pattern of tobacco use leading to clinically significant impairment or distress as manifested by at least <u>two</u> of the following in a 12-month period.

   i. Using tobacco in larger amounts or over a longer period than intended: *When you use tobacco, do you find that you use more, or for a longer time, than you planned to?*

ii. Persistent desire or unsuccessful effort to reduce tobacco use: *Do you want to cut back or stop using tobacco? Have you ever tried and failed to cut back or stop using tobacco?*

iii. Great deal of time spent: *Do you spend a great deal of your time obtaining tobacco, using tobacco, or recovering from your tobacco use?*

iv. Cravings: *Do you experience strong cravings for or desires to use tobacco?*

v. Failure to fulfill major role obligations: *Have you repeatedly failed to fulfill major obligations at work or home because of your tobacco use?*

vi. Continued use despite awareness of interpersonal or social problems: *Do you use tobacco even though you suspect, or even know, that your use creates or worsens interpersonal or social problems?*

vii. Giving up activities for tobacco: *Are there important social, occupational, or recreational activities that you have given up or reduced because of your tobacco use?*

viii. Use in hazardous situations: *Have you repeatedly used tobacco in situations in which use could be physically hazardous, such as smoking in bed?*

ix. Continued use despite awareness of physical or psychological problems: *Do you use tobacco even though you suspect, or even know, that your use creates or worsens problems with your mind and body?*

x. Tolerance as manifested by <u>either</u> of the following.

- Markedly increased amounts: *Do you find that in order to get the desired effect of tobacco, you need much more than you used to?*
- Markedly diminished effects: *If you use the same amount of tobacco as you used to, do you find that it has a lot less effect on you than it used to?*

xi. Withdrawal as manifested by <u>either</u> of the following.

- Characteristic tobacco withdrawal syndrome: *When you stop using tobacco, do you undergo withdrawal?*
- The same substance is taken to relieve or avoid withdrawal symptoms: *Have you ever used tobacco to avoid or relieve symptoms of tobacco withdrawal?*

b. Modifiers

　i. Specifiers
　　• In early remission
　　• In sustained remission
　　• On maintenance therapy
　　• In a controlled environment

　ii. Severity
　　• Mild [Z72.0, 572]: Two or three symptoms are present.
　　• Moderate [F17.200, 572]: Four or five symptoms are present.
　　• Severe [F17.200, 572]: Six or more symptoms are present.

c. Alternative: If a person experiences clinically significant problems associated with the use of tobacco that do not meet criteria for a specific diagnosis, consider unspecified tobacco-related disorder [F17.209, 577].

23. Tobacco Withdrawal [F17.203, 575–576]

a. Inclusion: Requires at least <u>four</u> of the following signs or symptoms developing within 24 hours of ceasing (or reducing) tobacco use that has been daily for at least several weeks.

　i. Irritability, frustration, or anger: *Over the past 24 hours, have you felt more irritable, frustrated, or angry than usual?*

　ii. Anxiety: *Over the past 24 hours, have you felt more worried or anxious than usual?*

　iii. Difficulty concentrating: *Over the past 24 hours, have you had difficulty staying focused on a task or activity?*

　iv. Increased appetite: *Over the past 24 hours, have you desired food more than usual?*

　v. Restlessness: *Over the past 24 hours, have you felt less able to remain at rest than usual?*

　vi. Depressed mood: *Over the past 24 hours, have you been feeling more down or depressed than usual?*

　vii. Insomnia: *Over the past 24 hours, have you found it more difficult than usual to get to sleep and to stay asleep?*

b. Exclusion: If the symptoms are attributable to another medical condition or are better explained by another mental disorder, including intoxication with or withdrawal from another substance, do not use this diagnosis.

24. Other (or Unknown) Substance Use Disorder [F19.x0, 577–580]

   a. Inclusion: Requires a problematic pattern of use of an intoxicating substance not able to be classified within the other substance categories listed previously, leading to clinically significant impairment or distress as manifested by at least <u>two</u> of the following in a 12-month period.

      i. Taking the substance in larger amounts or over a longer period than intended: *When you use the substance, do you find that you use it more often, or for a longer time, than you planned to?*

      ii. Persistent desire or unsuccessful effort to reduce substance use: *Do you want to cut back or stop using the substance? Have you ever tried and failed to cut back or stop using the substance?*

      iii. Great deal of time spent: *Do you spend a great deal of your time obtaining the substance, using the substance, or recovering from your substance use?*

      iv. Cravings: *Do you experience strong cravings for or desires to use the substance?*

      v. Failure to fulfill major role obligations: *Have you repeatedly failed to fulfill major obligations at work or home because of your substance use?*

      vi. Continued use despite awareness of interpersonal or social problems: *Do you use the substance even though you suspect, or even know, that your use creates or worsens interpersonal or social problems?*

      vii. Giving up activities for the substance: *Are there important social, occupational, or recreational activities that you have given up or reduced because of your substance use?*

      viii. Use in hazardous situations: *Have you repeatedly used the substance in situations in which use could be physically hazardous, such as driving a car or operating a machine?*

      ix. Continued use despite awareness of physical or psychological problems: *Do you use the substance even though you suspect, or even know, that your use creates or worsens problems with your mind and body?*

x.   Tolerance as manifested by either of the following.

- Markedly increased amounts: *Do you find that in order to get intoxicated or achieve the desired effect of substance use, you need much more than you used to?*
- Markedly diminished effects: *If you use the same amount of the substance as you used to, do you find that it has a lot less effect on you than it used to?*

xi. Withdrawal as manifested by either of the following.

- Characteristic withdrawal syndrome for the substance: *When you stop using the substance, do you undergo withdrawal?*
- The same or a closely related substance is taken to relieve or avoid withdrawal symptoms: *Have you ever taken the substance or another substance to prevent withdrawal?*

b. Modifiers

i. Specifiers

- In early remission
- In sustained remission
- In a controlled environment

ii. Severity

- Mild [F19.10, 578]: Two or three symptoms are present.
- Moderate [F19.20, 578]: Four or five symptoms are present.
- Severe [F19.20, 578]: Six or more symptoms are present.

25. Other (or Unknown) Substance Intoxication [F19.x29, 581–582]

a. Inclusion: Development of a reversible substance-specific syndrome attributable to recent ingestion of (or exposure to) a substance that is not listed elsewhere or is unknown.

b. Inclusion: Requires clinically significant problematic behavioral or psychological changes. *Since you began using this substance, have you observed any significant changes in your mood, judgment, ability to interact with others, or sense of time? Have you engaged in problematic activities or thought problematic thoughts that you would not have without this substance?*

c. Exclusion: If the symptoms are attributable to another medical condition or are better explained by another mental disorder, including intoxication with another substance, do not use this diagnosis.

26. Other (or Unknown) Substance Withdrawal [F19.239, 583–584]

   a. Inclusion: Development of a substance-specific syndrome shortly after the cessation of (or reduction in) use of the substance that has been heavy and prolonged.

   b. Inclusion: Requires clinically significant distress or impairment in social, occupational, or other important areas of functioning.

   c. Exclusion: If the symptoms are attributable to another medical condition or are better explained by another mental disorder, including withdrawal from another substance, do not use this diagnosis.

27. Gambling Disorder [F63.0, 585–589]

   a. Inclusion: Requires persistent, recurrent problematic gambling that leads to clinically significant impairment or distress, lasting at least 12 months, as indicated by at least <u>four</u> of the following symptoms.

      i. Escalates spending on gambling: *Do you find that it takes increasing amounts of money to get the excitement you want from gambling?*

      ii. Is irritable when quitting: *When you try to reduce or quit gambling, are you irritable or restless?*

      iii. Is unable to quit: *Have you unsuccessfully tried to reduce or quit gambling on several occasions?*

      iv. Is preoccupied: *Are you preoccupied with gambling?*

      v. Gambles when distressed: *When you are feeling anxious, down, or helpless, do you gamble?*

      vi. Chases losses: *After you lose money, do you return another day to try to get even?*

      vii. Lies: *Do you lie to conceal how much you gamble?*

      viii. Loses relationships: *Have you lost a relationship, job, or opportunity because of your gambling?*

      ix. Borrows money: *Do you have to rely on other people for money to cover desperate financial situations caused by gambling?*

   b. Exclusion: If the gambling behavior is better accounted for by a manic episode, do not use this diagnosis.

c. Modifiers

   i. Course

   - Episodic: Meeting diagnostic criteria at more than one time point, with symptoms subsiding between periods of gambling disorder for at least several months
   - Persistent: Experiencing continuous symptoms, to meet diagnostic criteria for multiple years
   - In early remission
   - In sustained remission

   ii. Severity

   - Mild: Four or five symptoms are present
   - Moderate: Six or seven symptoms are present
   - Severe: Eight or nine symptoms are present

Neurocognitive Disorders

DSM-5 pp. 591–643

Screening questions: *Have you had any problems with your concentration or memory? Can you help me understand the extent to which you might be having these difficulties?*

If yes, ask: *Did these experiences ever cause you significant trouble with your friends or family, at work, or in another setting?*

- If a person is disoriented, proceed to delirium criteria.
- If a person is oriented but experiencing cognitive difficulties, ask: *Are you able to live as independently as you used to? For example, can you cook and keep track of your medications and your finances like you used to?*

  - If a person answers yes, proceed to mild neurocognitive disorder criteria.
  - If a person or her caregiver answers no, proceed to major neurocognitive disorder criteria.

1. Delirium [F1x.x21, 596–601]

   a. Inclusion: Requires the presence of <u>all three</u> of the following disturbances, which are usually assessed through examination, especially the Mini-Mental

State Examination (MMSE), rather than through diagnostic questions.

   i. Disturbance in attention and awareness, as manifested by reduced ability to direct, focus, sustain, and shift attention.
   ii. Disturbance that represents an acute change from baseline, developed over a short period of time (hours to days), with severity that tends to fluctuate during the course of a day.
   iii. Change in cognition, such as memory deficit, disorientation, language disturbance, visuospatial ability, or perception.

b. Exclusions

   i. If the change in cognition is better accounted for by a preexisting, established, or evolving neurocognitive disorder, do not use this diagnosis.
   ii. If the disturbance in cognition occurs in the context of a severely reduced level of arousal, such as coma, do not use this diagnosis.
   iii. If the disturbance in cognition is a direct physiological consequence of another medical condition, substance intoxication or withdrawal, or exposure to a toxin or is due to multiple etiologies, do not use this diagnosis.

c. Modifiers

   i. Subtypes

      • Substance intoxication delirium [F1x.x21, 596]: Use instead of substance intoxication when inclusion criteria i and iii above predominate in the clinical picture.
      • Substance withdrawal delirium [F1x.23x, 597]: Use instead of substance withdrawal when inclusion criteria i and iii above predominate in the clinical picture.
      • Medication-induced delirium [F1x.921, 597]: Use when inclusion criteria i and iii arise as a side effect of a medication taken as prescribed.
      • Delirium due to another medical condition [F05, 597]
      • Delirium due to multiple etiologies [F05, 597]

ii. Specifiers
- Course
  - Acute: Lasting a few hours or days
  - Persistent: Lasting weeks or months
- Descriptive features
  - Hyperactive
  - Hypoactive
  - Mixed level of activity

d. Alternatives: If you are unable to determine why a person is experiencing delirium or if the delirium is subsyndromal, consider unspecified delirium [R41.0, 602]. If you wish to communicate the specific reason a person's symptoms do not meet full criteria for delirium, consider other specified delirium [R41.0, 602]. An example is attenuated delirium syndrome.

2. Mild Neurocognitive Disorder [G31.84, 602–611]

a. Inclusion: Requires evidence of modest cognitive decline from a previous level of performance in one or more cognitive domains (complex attention, executive function, learning and memory, language, perceptual-motor, or social cognition) based on both of the following, which are usually assessed through examination, especially the MMSE, rather than through diagnostic questions.

i. Concern of the person, a knowledgeable informant, or the practitioner that a significant cognitive decline has occurred

ii. A modest impairment in cognitive performance, preferably documented by standardized neuropsychological testing or, in its absence, another quantified clinical assessment

b. Inclusion: The cognitive deficits do not interfere with capacity for independence in everyday activities, although greater effort, compensatory strategies, or accommodation may be required.

c. Exclusion: If the cognitive impairments occur exclusively in the context of a delirium or are primarily the result of another mental disorder, do not use this diagnosis.

    d. Modifiers

        i. Subtypes (see full descriptions in "Major Neuro-cognitive Disorders" section, below)

- Alzheimer's disease [G31.84, 611–614]
- Frontotemporal lobar degeneration [G31.84, 614–618]
- Lewy body disease [G31.84, 618–621]
- Vascular disease [G31.84, 621–624]
- Traumatic brain injury [G31.84, 624–627]
- Substance/medication use [F1x.xxx, 627–632]
- HIV infection [G31.84, 632–634]
- Prion disease [G31.84, 634–636]
- Parkinson's disease [G31.84, 636–638]
- Huntington's disease [G31.84, 638–641]
- Another medical condition [G31.84, 641–642]
- Multiple etiologies [G31.84, 642–643]
- Unspecified [R41.9, 643]

        ii. Specifiers

- Without behavioral disturbance
- With behavioral disturbance

3. Major Neurocognitive Disorder [probable 29x.xx, possible 331.9, 602–611]

    a. Inclusion: Requires evidence of significant cognitive decline from a previous level of performance in one or more cognitive domains (complex attention, executive function, learning and memory, language, perceptual-motor, or social cognition) based on both of the following, which are usually assessed through examination, especially the MMSE, rather than through diagnostic questions.

        i. Concern of the person, a knowledgeable informant, or the practitioner, that a significant cognitive decline has occurred.

        ii. A substantial impairment in cognitive performance, preferably documented by standardized neuropsychological testing or, in its absence, another quantified clinical assessment.

    b. Inclusion: The cognitive deficits interfere with independence in everyday activities.

    c. Exclusions: If the cognitive impairments occur exclusively in the context of a delirium or are primarily the result of another mental disorder, do not use this diagnosis.

d. Modifiers

  i. Subtypes

- Alzheimer's disease [probable F02.8x, possible G31.9, 611–614]: Characteristically associated with an insidious onset and gradual progression, in which decline in memory and learning is an early and prominent feature. Requires exclusion of cerebrovascular disease; another neurodegenerative disease; the effects of a substance; or another mental, neurological, or systemic disorder.

- Frontotemporal lobar degeneration [probable F02.8x, possible G31.9, 614–618]: Requires evidence for the characteristic impairments associated with behavioral or language variants. The behavioral variant can include prominent decline in social cognition and/or executive abilities; behavioral disinhibition; apathy or inertia; loss of sympathy or empathy; perseverative, stereotyped, or compulsive/ritualistic behavior; and hyperorality and dietary changes. The language variant includes prominent decline in language ability in the form of speech production, word finding, object naming, grammar, or word comprehension. In both variants, learning, memory, and perceptual-motor function are relatively spared. Requires the exclusion of cerebrovascular disease; another neurodegenerative disease; the effects of a substance; or another mental, neurological, or systemic disorder.

- Lewy body disease [probable F02.8x, possible G31.9, 618–621]: Requires evidence of fluctuating cognition with pronounced variations in attention and alertness; recurrent visual hallucinations that are typically well formed and detailed; and spontaneous features of parkinsonism, with onset of motor symptoms subsequent to the cognitive impairment. Requires the exclusion of cerebrovascular disease; another neurodegenerative disease; the effects of a substance; or another mental, neurological, or systemic disorder.

- Vascular disease [probable F01.5x, possible G31.9, 621–624]: Requires evidence of cerebrovascular disease and exclusion of other known neurocognitive disorders. Deficits in complex attention (including the speed of information processing) and frontal-executive function are characteristic. Onset is temporally related to one or more cerebrovascular events. Requires the exclusion of another brain disease or systemic disorder.
- Traumatic brain injury [F02.8x, 624–627]: Requires an impact to the head or other rapid displacement of the brain within the skull that results in one or more of the following: loss of consciousness, posttraumatic amnesia, disorientation and confusion, or neurological signs. The cognitive deficits present immediately following the injury or after recovery of consciousness and persist past the acute postinjury period (i.e., for at least 1 week).
- Substance/medication-induced [F1x.xxx, 627–632]: Requires presumptive evidence of an etiological relationship between past or present substance use and cognitive deficits. A person must have used a substance or medication for a duration and extent capable of producing the neurocognitive impairment. Requires the exclusion of another medical condition or mental disorder or current intoxication or withdrawal.
- HIV infection [F02.8x, 632–634]: Requires documented infection with HIV. Symptoms cannot be better explained by secondary brain diseases such as progressive multifocal leukoencephalopathy or cryptococcal meningitis. Requires the exclusion of another medical condition or mental disorder.
- Prion disease [F02.8x, 634–636]: Requires evidence that the neurocognitive disorder is due to a prion disease. Requires the presence of motor features of prion disease, such as myoclonus or ataxia, or biomarker evidence. Requires the exclusion of another medical condition or mental disorder.

- Parkinson's disease [probable F02.8x, possible G31.9, 636–638]: Requires the established presence of Parkinson's disease and the insidious onset and gradual progression of impairing cognitive deficits. Requires the exclusion of another medical condition or mental disorder.
- Huntington's disease [F02.8x, 638–641]: Requires the presence of clinically established Huntington's disease or evidence of risk for the disease based on family history or genetic testing and the insidious onset and gradual progression of impairing cognitive deficits. Requires the exclusion of another medical condition or mental disorder.
- Another medical condition [F02.8x, 641–642]: Requires evidence that the neurocognitive disorder is due to another medical condition. Requires the exclusion of cognitive deficits due to another mental disorder or specific neurocognitive disorder.
- Multiple etiologies [F02.8x, 642–643]: Requires evidence from the history, physical examination, or laboratory findings that the neurocognitive disorder is the pathophysiological consequence of more than one etiological process, excluding substances. Requires the exclusion of cognitive deficits due to delirium or another mental disorder.
- Unspecified [R41.9, 643]: Can be used in the event of a subthreshold syndrome, an atypical presentation, an uncertain etiology, or a specific syndrome not listed in DSM-5.

ii. Specifiers

- Without behavioral disturbance
- With behavioral disturbance

iii. Severity

- Mild: Difficulties with instrumental activities of daily living
- Moderate: Difficulties with basic activities of daily living
- Severe: Fully dependent

Personality Disorders

DSM-5 pp. 645–684

Screening question: *When people reflect on their life, they can often identify patterns—characteristic thoughts, moods, and actions—that began when they were young and have since continued to occur in many personal and social situations. Thinking about your own life, can you identify any such patterns that have caused significant problems with your friends or family, at work, or in another setting?*

If yes, ask: *When you think about these characteristic patterns of behavior that began when you were a young person, can you recognize enduring patterns in how you perceive and interpret yourself, other people, and events; how you respond emotionally to exciting or difficult circumstances; how you interact with other people; or how well you control your impulses and urges?*

If yes, ask: *When you look over your life, can you see that one or more of the following ways of being has been relatively stable over time?*

- *Distrusting other people and suspecting them of being mean.* If distrust and suspiciousness of others predominate, proceed to paranoid personality disorder criteria.
- *Feeling disconnected from close relationships and preferring not to express much emotion.* If detachment and restricted range of emotions predominate, proceed to schizoid personality disorder criteria.
- *Feeling uncomfortable in close relationships and preferring activities that many other people consider unusual or eccentric.* If discomfort in close relationships and eccentric behavior predominate, proceed to schizotypal personality disorder criteria.
- *Disregarding the rights of other people without concern for how it affects them.* If disregard for the rights of other people predominates, proceed to antisocial personality disorder criteria.
- *Experiencing yourself, your mood, and your relationships as constantly changing.* If instability in relationships, self-image, and affects predominates, proceed to borderline personality disorder criteria.
- *Being more emotional and desiring more attention than other people.* If excessive emotionality and attention seeking pre-

dominate, proceed to histrionic personality disorder criteria.

- *Sensing that you are much more accomplished or deserving than other people.* If grandiosity and need for admiration predominate, proceed to narcissistic personality disorder criteria.

- *Avoiding other people because you feel inferior or fear they will criticize or reject you.* If social inhibition and feelings of inadequacy predominate, proceed to avoidant personality disorder criteria.

- *Wanting so much for someone to take care of you that you become submissive or clingy and repeatedly fear they will separate from you.* If a need to be taken care of predominates, proceed to dependent personality disorder criteria.

- *Focusing on getting things rightly ordered, perfect, or under control.* If preoccupation with orderliness, perfectionism, and control predominates, proceed to obsessive-compulsive personality disorder criteria.

1. Paranoid Personality Disorder [F60.0, 649–652]

    a. Inclusion: Requires a pervasive pattern of distrust and suspiciousness of others such that their motives are interpreted as malevolent, as indicated by at least <u>four</u> of the following manifestations.

        i. Suspects exploitation, harm, or deception: *Do you frequently suspect that other people are exploiting, harming, or deceiving you, even when you have limited evidence for these suspicions?*

        ii. Is preoccupied with doubts: *Do you find that thinking about whether the people in your life are loyal or trustworthy dominates your thoughts?*

        iii. Is reluctant to confide: *Are you often reluctant to tell people about a personal or private matter because you fear they will use the information to harm you?*

        iv. Reads hidden meanings: *Do other people often say things or do things that you think are demeaning or threatening to you?*

        v. Persistently bears grudges: *When someone insults, injures, or slights you, do you find it very hard to forgive? Do you usually bear grudges?*

        vi. Perceives character attacks: *Do you find that other people often say or do things to attack your character or reputation? Do you counterattack or react angrily?*

vii. Suspects infidelity: *When you are involved in a relationship, do you repeatedly suspect your partner of being unfaithful to you, without having any evidence?*

b. Exclusion: If the disturbance occurs exclusively in the course of a psychotic disorder or a bipolar or depressive disorder with psychotic features or is a physiological effect of another medical condition, do not use this diagnosis.

2. Schizoid Personality Disorder [F60.1, 652–655]

a. Inclusion: Requires a pervasive pattern of detachment from social relationships and a restricted range of expression of emotions in interpersonal settings, as indicated by at least <u>four</u> of the following manifestations.

i. Neither desires nor enjoys close relationships: *Do you find that you neither desire to be close to nor enjoy being close to other people, including your family?*

ii. Chooses solitary activities: *When you have a choice, do you almost always choose activities that you can do alone, without other people?*

iii. Has little interest in sexual experiences with others: *Would it be OK with you if you lived the rest of your life without romantic or sexual experiences with other people?*

iv. Takes pleasure in few activities: *Do you find that very few activities bring you pleasure or enjoyment?*

v. Lacks close friends and confidants: *Other than your immediate family, do you find that you do not have close friends or people with whom you share personal matters or secrets?*

vi. Appears indifferent to praise or criticism: *When other people praise or criticize you, do you find that it does not affect you?*

vii. Shows emotional coldness or detachment: *Do you rarely experience strong emotions such as anger or joy? Do you rarely reciprocate gestures or facial expressions such as smiles or nods?*

b. Exclusion: If the disturbance occurs exclusively in the course of a psychotic disorder, a bipolar or depressive disorder with psychotic features, or autism spectrum disorder or is a physiological effect of another medical condition, do not use this diagnosis.

3. Schizotypal Personality Disorder [F21, 655–659]

   a. Inclusion: Requires a pervasive pattern of social and interpersonal deficits marked by acute discomfort with and reduced capacity for close relationships as well as by cognitive or perceptual distortions or eccentricities of behavior, as indicated by at least <u>five</u> of the following manifestations.

      i. Ideas of reference: *Does it often feel as though other people are talking about you or watching you?*

      ii. Odd beliefs or magical thinking: *Are you very superstitious? Are you preoccupied with paranormal or magical phenomena? Do you have special powers to sense events before they happen or to read the thoughts of other people?*

      iii. Unusual perceptual experiences: *Do you sometimes have the sense that another person others cannot see is present and speaking with you?*

      iv. Odd thinking and speech: *Do other people ever tell you that the things you say, or the way you say them, are unusual or even inappropriate?*

      v. Suspiciousness or paranoia: *Do you frequently suspect that other people are exploiting, harming, or deceiving you?*

      vi. Inappropriate or constricted affect: *Do you notice that your emotional experiences and expressions stay within a narrow range and do not change much over time? Have other people told you that you do not respond to emotionally provocative situations as they would expect you to?*

      vii. Odd or eccentric appearance or behavior: *Do other people ever respond to you as if your behavior or appearance is odd or bizarre?*

      viii. Lack of close friends and confidants: *Other than your immediate family, do you find that you do not have close friends or people with whom you share personal matters or secrets?*

      ix. Excessive social anxiety: *Are you usually worried or anxious in social settings, especially when around unfamiliar people?*

   b. Exclusion: If the disturbance occurs exclusively in the course of a psychotic disorder, a bipolar or depressive disorder with psychotic features, or autism spectrum disorder, do not use this diagnosis.

4. Antisocial Personality Disorder [F60.2, 659–663]

   a. Inclusion: Requires a pervasive pattern of disregard for and violation of the rights of others, as indicated by at least <u>three</u> of the following manifestations.

      i. Repeated performance of acts that are grounds for arrest: *Have you repeatedly destroyed or stolen the property of other people, harassed other people, or done other things that could have gotten you arrested?*

      ii. Deceitfulness: *Do you often misrepresent yourself by claiming accomplishments, qualities, or identities that are not your own? Do you often deceive other people for pleasure or financial gain?*

      iii. Impulsivity: *Do you often struggle to formulate and follow a plan? Do you often act on the spur of the moment, without a plan or consideration of the consequences?*

      iv. Aggressiveness resulting in assaults: *Are you often so grumpy or irritable that you frequently confront or even attack other people? Have you ever attacked someone or been in physical fights that did not begin as self-defense?*

      v. Reckless disregard for safety: *Do you often engage in dangerous, risky, and potentially self-damaging activities with little thought about the consequences for yourself or others?*

      vi. Consistent irresponsibility: *When you enter into agreements or make promises, do you often disregard and fail to follow through on your commitments? When you have familial obligations and financial debts, do you often disregard them?*

      vii. Lack of remorse: *Are you rarely concerned about the feelings, needs, or suffering of other people? If you have ever hurt or mistreated someone else, did you feel very little regret or remorse after doing so?*

   b. Inclusion: Evidence of conduct disorder with onset before age 15 years.

   c. Exclusion: If the disturbance occurs exclusively in the course of a psychotic or bipolar disorder, do not use this diagnosis.

5. Borderline Personality Disorder [F60.3, 663–666]

   a. Inclusion: Requires a pervasive pattern of instability of interpersonal relationships, self-image, and affects and marked impulsivity, as indicated by at least <u>five</u> of the following manifestations.

i. Frantic efforts to avoid abandonment: *When you sense that someone close to you is going to abandon you, do you undertake emotional or even frantic efforts to keep them from leaving?*

ii. Unstable interpersonal relationships: *Are most of your close relationships intense and unstable? Do you alternate between feelings that the people in your life are really good and really bad?*

iii. Identity disturbance: *Do you have a very unstable or poorly developed sense of who you are? Do your aspirations, goals, opinions, and values change suddenly and frequently?*

iv. Self-damaging impulsivity in at least two areas that are not suicidal or self-mutilating behavior (e.g., spending, sex, substance abuse, reckless driving, binge eating): *Do you often act on the spur of the moment, without a plan or consideration for the outcome? Do you frequently engage in dangerous, risky, and potentially self-damaging activities without regard to their consequences?*

v. Parasuicidal or suicidal behavior: *Do you frequently threaten to harm yourself or even kill yourself? Have you made recurrent attempts to hurt, harm, or kill yourself?*

vi. Affective instability: *Are your emotions easily aroused or intense? Do you often have intense feelings of sadness, annoyance, or worry that last usually only a few hours and never more than a few days?*

vii. Chronic emptiness: *Do you chronically feel empty?*

viii. Anger: *Do you often experience intense anger much stronger than is called for by the event or circumstance that triggered it, and do you frequently lose your temper?*

ix. Transient paranoia or dissociation: *At times of stress, do you ever feel that other people are conspiring against you or that you are an outside observer of your own mind, thoughts, feelings, and body?*

6. Histrionic Personality Disorder [F60.4, 667–669]

a. Inclusion: Requires a pervasive pattern of excessive emotionality and attention seeking, as indicated by at least <u>five</u> of the following manifestations.

i. Is uncomfortable when not the center of attention: *Do you usually feel uncomfortable or unappreciated when you are not the center of attention?*

ii. Demonstrates seductive or provocative behavior: *Do you flirt with most of the people you meet, even if you are not attracted to them?*

iii. Displays shifting and shallow emotions: *When you express emotions or feelings, do they change rapidly? Have other people told you that your emotions seem to have little depth or to be insincere?*

iv. Uses appearance to draw attention: *Do you usually "dress to impress," spending your time and energy on your clothes and appearance so you can draw attention to yourself?*

v. Has impressionistic and vague speech: *Do other people ever tell you that you have strong opinions but that they find it hard to understand the underlying reasons for your opinions?*

vi. Displays dramatic or exaggerated emotions: *Are you a very expressive or even dramatic person? Have your friends or family repeatedly told you that you embarrassed them with your public displays of emotion?*

vii. Is suggestible: *Do you frequently change your opinions and feelings based on the people around you or the people you admire?*

viii. Considers relationships more intimate than they are: *Do you often feel close to people early in a relationship and share personal details of your life? Have you been hurt by relationships that you thought were more serious or intimate than the other person did?*

7. Narcissistic Personality Disorder [F60.81, 669–672]

   a. Inclusion: Requires a pervasive pattern of grandiosity (in fantasy or behavior), need for admiration, and lack of empathy, as indicated by at least <u>five</u> of the following manifestations.

      i. Has grandiose sense of self-importance: *Would you describe yourself and your accomplishments as so special and unique that they set you apart from your peers?*

      ii. Is preoccupied with fantasies of unlimited success: *When you imagine the life of your dreams, do you think a lot about having unlimited success, limitless power, unparalleled brilliance, remarkable beauty, or supreme love?*

      iii. Expects to be affiliated with high-status people or institutions: *Are your abilities and needs so special that you feel as though you should associate only with gifted people or institutions? Do you feel that only unique or gifted people are capable of understanding you?*

      iv. Requires excessive admiration: *Do you often feel offended if people you respect do not give you the admiration you deserve?*

      v. Has sense of entitlement: *Do you often get annoyed or irritated when people do not follow your wishes or treat you the way you deserve?*

      vi. Is exploitative: *Are you good at getting people to do what you want? Do you ever take advantage of people to get the resources or privileges you deserve?*

      vii. Lacks empathy: *Do you find it hard to recognize or identify with the feelings and needs of other people?*

      viii. Is envious or expects others to be envious: *Do other people really envy you or your life? Do you spend a lot of time envying other people or their lives?*

      ix. Demonstrates arrogant behaviors or attitudes: *Have other people ever told you that you act in haughty, patronizing, or arrogant ways?*

8. Avoidant Personality Disorder [F60.6, 672–675]

    a. Inclusion: Requires a pervasive pattern of social inhibition, feelings of inadequacy, and hypersensitivity to negative evaluations, as indicated by at least <u>four</u> of the following manifestations.

      i. Avoids occupational activities involving interpersonal contact: *Do you often avoid activities that involve a lot of contact with other people because you fear they will criticize or reject you?*

      ii. Needs assurance before getting involved with other people: *Do you avoid making new friends unless you are certain they like you and accept you without criticism?*

      iii. Is restrained in intimate relationships because of fear of being shamed: *In your close relationships, are you usually cautious or restrained because you fear being shamed or ridiculed?*

      iv. Is preoccupied with criticism in social situations: *In social situations, do you spend a great deal of time worrying that other people will criticize or reject you?*

v. Has feelings of inadequacy that inhibit interpersonal situations: *In new relationships, are you usually shy, quiet, or inhibited because you fear that other people will find you inadequate or unsuitable?*

vi. Has negative self-perception: *Do you perceive yourself to be socially inept, personally unappealing, or inferior to others?*

vii. Is reluctant to take risks: *Are you usually reluctant to take personal risks or to engage in new activities because you fear you will be embarrassed?*

9. Dependent Personality Disorder [F60.7, 675–678]

a. Inclusion: Requires a pervasive and excessive need to be taken care of that leads to submissive, clinging behavior and fear of separation, as indicated by at least <u>five</u> of the following manifestations.

i. Struggles to make everyday decisions without reassurance: *Do you struggle to make everyday decisions, such as what to eat or wear, without advice and reassurance from other people?*

ii. Needs others to assume responsibility: *Do you prefer to let someone else take responsibility for the major decisions in your life, such as where to live, what kind of work you do, and who you befriend?*

iii. Has difficulty disagreeing: *Do you find it really hard to disagree with the people you count on because you fear they will disapprove or withdraw their support?*

iv. Struggles to initiate: *Do you usually lack the self-confidence to start a new project or do things independently?*

v. Goes to excessive lengths to obtain support: *Do you go to great lengths to receive care and support from other people, even volunteering to do things that you find unpleasant?*

vi. Feels helpless when alone: *When you are alone, do you often feel uncomfortable or even helpless because you fear being unable to care for yourself?*

vii. Urgently seeks relationships: *After a close relationship ends, do you urgently seek another relationship in which you can receive the care and support you need?*

viii. Is preoccupied with fear of being alone: *Do you spend a great deal of time worrying about being left alone with no one to care for you?*

10. Obsessive-Compulsive Personality Disorder [F60.5, 678–682]

a. Inclusion: Requires a pervasive pattern of preoccupation with orderliness, perfectionism, and mental and interpersonal control, at the expense of flexibility, openness, and efficiency, as indicated by at least <u>four</u> of the following manifestations.

i. Preoccupation with order interferes with the point of the activity: *Do you often find that you are so focused on the details, rules, lists, order, organization, or schedules for an activity that you lose the essential point of the activity?*

ii. Perfectionism interferes with task completion: *Are you often unable to complete projects because you cannot meet the high standards you set for yourself?*

iii. Devotion to work at the expense of friendships: *Do you devote so much time and energy to your work that you have little time for friendships or recreational activities? When you do participate in recreational activities, do you approach them as serious tasks that require organization and mastery?*

iv. Scrupulousness: *Do other people who share your cultural or religious identification ever tell you that they find you too strict or too concerned with not doing something wrong? Do you aspire to moral standards that are so high that it is difficult for you to realize your goals?*

v. Inability to discard worn-out objects: *Do you often find it hard to discard worn-out or worthless objects even when they have no sentimental value?*

vi. Reluctance to give up control of tasks: *Do you find it hard to work with other people or delegate tasks because you fear they will not do things the way you would?*

vii. Miserliness: *Do you usually find it hard to spend money on yourself or other people? Do you maintain a standard of living well below what you can afford in an effort to save money for a catastrophe?*

viii. Rigidity: *Does your need to be right or to not change your position frequently make it difficult to make and maintain relationships with other people?*

11. Alternatives

a. If a person exhibits a persistent personality disturbance that represents a change from her previous characteristic personality pattern and there is evidence that the disturbance is the direct consequence of another medical condition, consider personality change due to another medical condition [F07.0, 682–684]. If the diagnosis is better explained by another mental disorder, occurs exclusively during an episode of delirium, or does not cause clinically significant distress or impairment, do not use this diagnosis.

b. If a person exhibits symptoms characteristic of a personality disorder that cause clinically significant distress or impairment but do not meet full criteria for a specific personality disorder, consider unspecified personality disorder [F60.9, 684]. If you wish to communicate the specific reason that the presentation does not meet the criteria for a specific personality disorder, consider other specified personality disorder [F60.89, 684].

Other Conditions That May Be a Focus of Clinical Attention

DSM-5 pp. 715–727

DSM-5 includes other conditions and problems that may be a focus of clinical attention or that may otherwise affect the diagnosis, course, prognosis, or treatment of a patient's mental disorder. These include, but are not limited to, the psychosocial and environmental problems that were coded on Axis IV in DSM-IV-TR (American Psychiatric Association 2000). The authors of DSM-5 provide a selected list of conditions and problems drawn from ICD-10-CM (most have Z codes). These conditions or problems may be coded if they are the reason for the current encounter or they help to explain the need for a test, procedure, or treatment.

Conditions and problems from this list may also be included in the medical record as useful information about circumstances that may affect the patient's care, regardless of their relevance to the current visit. The conditions and problems listed in this section are not mental disorders. Their inclusion in DSM-5 is meant to draw attention to the scope of additional issues encountered in routine clinical practice and to provide a systematic listing that may be useful to clinicians in documenting these issues.

In Chapter 12, "Rating Scales and Alternative Diagnostic Systems," we include a list of ICD-10-CM Z codes that are commonly used in elder mental health.

CHAPTER 8

A Brief Version of DSM-5

TABLE 8–1. Abbreviated DSM-5 criteria for common diagnoses among older adults

Diagnosis	Symptoms	Criteria/time
Schizophrenia spectrum and other psychotic disorders		
Schizophrenia	Delusions	≥2 for ≥1 month *AND*
	Hallucinations	
	Disorganized speech	
	Grossly disorganized or catatonic behavior	
	Negative symptoms	
	(At least one symptom must be delusions, hallucinations, or disorganized speech)	
	Continuous signs of disturbance	≥6 months
Schizoaffective disorder	Delusions	≥2 for ≥1 month *AND*
	Hallucinations	
	Disorganized speech	
	Grossly disorganized or catatonic behavior	
	Negative symptoms	
	(At least one symptom must be delusions, hallucinations, or disorganized speech)	
	Major depressive or manic episodes	≥50% of the time *AND*

TABLE 8–1. Abbreviated DSM-5 criteria for common diagnoses among older adults *(continued)*

Diagnosis	Symptoms	Criteria/time
Schizoaffective disorder *(continued)*	Delusions or hallucinations without depressive or manic episodes	≥2 weeks
Bipolar and related disorders		
Bipolar I disorder	Persistently elevated or irritable mood Persistently increased goal-directed activity or energy	Both for ≥1 week (or any duration if hospitalized) *AND*
	Mania Inflated self-esteem or grandiosity Decreased need for sleep Pressured speech Racing thoughts or flight of ideas Distractibility Increased goal-directed activity or psychomotor agitation Risky behavior	≥3

TABLE 8–1. Abbreviated DSM-5 criteria for common diagnoses among older adults *(continued)*

Diagnosis	Symptoms	Criteria/time
Bipolar II disorder	Hypomania Inflated self-esteem or grandiosity Decreased need for sleep Pressured speech Racing thoughts Distractibility Increased goal-directed activity Risky behavior *without* psychosis or hospitalization	≥3 for ≥4 days
Depressive disorders		
Major depressive disorder	Depressed mood; loss of interest in activities or pleasure (anhedonia) Weight loss or decreased appetite Insomnia or hypersomnia Agitation or retardation Fatigue or loss of energy Feelings of worthlessness or excessive guilt Decreased ability to concentrate Thoughts of death or suicide	≥1 for ≥2 weeks *AND* ≥4 for ≥2 weeks

TABLE 8–1. Abbreviated DSM-5 criteria for common diagnoses among older adults *(continued)*

Diagnosis	Symptoms	Criteria/time
Persistent depressive disorder (dysthymia)	Depressed mood most of the day, more days than not	≥2 years *AND*
	Poor appetite or overeating	≥2
	Insomnia or hypersomnia	
	Low energy or fatigue	
	Low self-esteem	
	Poor concentration or difficulty making decisions	
	Feelings of hopelessness	
Anxiety disorders		
Panic disorder	Palpitations	≥4 *AND*
	Sweating	
	Trembling	
	Shortness of breath	
	Choking	
	Chest pain	
	Nausea or abdominal distress	
	Dizziness	
	Chills or heat sensations	
	Paresthesias	

TABLE 8–1. Abbreviated DSM-5 criteria for common diagnoses among older adults *(continued)*

Diagnosis	Symptoms	Criteria/time
Panic disorder *(continued)*	Derealization Fear of insanity Fear of death	
	Persistent concern or worry about attacks Significant behavior change related to attacks	≥1 for ≥1 month
Generalized anxiety disorder	Restlessness Easy fatigability Difficulty concentrating Irritability Muscle tension Sleep disturbance	≥3 for ≥6 months
Obsessive-compulsive and related disorders		
Obsessive-compulsive disorder	Obsessions: recurrent and intrusive thoughts, urges, or images that a person attempts to ignore or suppress through compulsive acts *AND/OR* Compulsions: repetitive behaviors or mental acts to reduce distress	≥1 hour/day

DSM-5® Pocket Guide for Elder Mental Health

TABLE 8–1. Abbreviated DSM-5 criteria for common diagnoses among older adults *(continued)*

Diagnosis	Symptoms	Criteria/time
Trauma- and stressor-related disorders		
Posttraumatic stress disorder	Exposure to trauma	
	Intrusive experiences	≥1 for ≥1 month *AND*
	Memories	
	Dreams	
	Flashbacks	
	Exposure distress	
	Physiological reactions	
	Avoiding	≥1 for ≥1 month *AND*
	Internal reminders	
	External reminders	

TABLE 8–1. Abbreviated DSM-5 criteria for common diagnoses among older adults *(continued)*

Diagnosis	Symptoms	Criteria/time
Posttraumatic stress disorder *(continued)*	Negative symptoms Impaired memories Negative self-image Blame Negative emotional states Decreased participation Detachment Inability to experience pleasure	≥2 for ≥1 month *AND*
	Arousal Irritability and angry outbursts Recklessness Hypervigilance Exaggerated startle Impaired concentration Sleep disturbance	≥2 for ≥1 month

DSM-5® Pocket Guide for Elder Mental Health

TABLE 8–1. Abbreviated DSM-5 criteria for common diagnoses among older adults *(continued)*

Diagnosis	Symptoms	Criteria/time
Somatic symptom and related disorders		
Somatic symptom disorder	Somatic symptom(s) that are distressing or that significantly disrupt daily life	≥6 months *AND*
	Excessive thoughts, feelings, or behaviors related to symptoms	≥1
	Disproportionate, persistent thoughts about the seriousness of symptoms	
	Persistently high anxiety about health or symptoms	
	Excessive time or energy devoted to health or symptoms	
Illness anxiety disorder	Preoccupation with being seriously ill	*ALL* for ≥6 months
	Absent or mild somatic symptoms	
	High anxiety about health	
	Excessive health-related behaviors	
Conversion disorder (functional neurological symptom disorder)	Symptom(s) of altered voluntary motor or sensory function	*BOTH*
	Clinical evidence of incompatibility between reported symptoms and known medical and neurological conditions	

TABLE 8-1. Abbreviated DSM-5 criteria for common diagnoses among older adults *(continued)*

Diagnosis	Symptoms	Criteria/time
Feeding and eating disorders		
Anorexia nervosa	Persistent energy intake restriction Intense fear of gaining weight or significant weight normalization–interfering behaviors Disturbance in self-perceived body shape or weight	*ALL*
Bulimia nervosa	Recurrent episodes of binge eating Recurrent inappropriate compensatory behaviors to prevent weight gain Self-evaluation unduly influenced by body shape and weight	Both binge eating and inappropriate compensatory behaviors occur at least weekly for ≥3 months
Sleep-wake disorders		
Insomnia disorder	Difficulty initiating sleep Difficulty maintaining sleep Early-morning awakening with inability to return to sleep	≥1 for ≥3 nights per week for ≥3 months *DESPITE* adequate opportunities for sleep

TABLE 8–1. Abbreviated DSM-5 criteria for common diagnoses among older adults *(continued)*

Diagnosis	Symptoms	Criteria/time
Neurocognitive disorders		
Delirium	Disturbance of consciousness; acute change from baseline, generally with fluctuating severity; cognitive change	Acute
Major neurocognitive disorder	Significant cognitive decline (≥2 standard deviations below normal) that interferes with independence	Insidious
Mild neurocognitive disorder	Mild cognitive decline (1–2 standard deviations below normal) that does not interfere with independence (but may require greater effort, compensatory strategies, or accommodations)	Insidious

Source. American Psychiatric Association 2013.

SECTION III

Additional Tools and Initial Treatments

CHAPTER 9

A Stepwise Approach to Differential Diagnosis

A good interviewer should consider as many diagnoses as possible while investigating the nature of a person's distress (Feinstein 1967). Although an entire manual (First 2014) has been designed specifically to teach the differential diagnosis for DSM-5 (American Psychiatric Association 2013), we provide in this chapter a general six-step approach to generating the differential diagnosis in older adults. As you develop your clinical decision-making skills, it will be helpful to follow these steps sequentially so you will consider each possible cause of mental distress.

Step 1: Consider to What Extent the Signs and Symptoms Are Related to a Stressor or Functional Change

Your thorough evaluation of an older adult should eventually include recommended health screening and some kind of functional assessment. Although formal assessments of physical health and functional ability are beyond the scope of this book, you should be aware of how normal aging affects balance, cognition, memory, smell, sleep, and vision. Remember that there can be significant differences between a patient's chronological age and her functional age. Function also depends on baseline ability, and a thorough social history imparts a sense of how a patient's current behavior relates to her usual behavior. Even in a brief interview, it is useful to observe how your patient communicates and behaves and to compare her communication and behavior with those appropriate for her age, culture, and education. If you observe a disjunction, consider these possibilities:

- The patient is having a transient response to a particular event. If distress or impairment develops as a maladaptive response to an identifiable psychosocial stressor, consider an adjustment disorder.
- The patient has an immature defense mechanism, which may indicate a personality trait or disorder.
- The patient is having a developmental conflict in a particular relationship.
- The patient is experiencing a change in functional ability.

Step 2: Consider to What Extent the Signs and Symptoms Are Related to a Caregiver Conflict

As human beings we are, in the words of the philosopher Alasdair MacIntyre (2012), "dependent rational animals" because we depend on "particular others for protection and sustenance" (p. 1). For older adults, aging can be experienced as a return to dependence after decades of perceived independence. Older adults depend on other people as caregivers. As you evaluate your patient, observe how she does (or does not) speak about her caregivers. As you observe, consider these possibilities:

- A caregiver and the patient have communication difficulties or cultural differences.
- A caregiver is a poor fit with the patient.
- A caregiver is abusing, neglecting, or otherwise harming the patient.
- A caregiver is experiencing mental distress, which results in the caregiver unintentionally worsening a patient's signs or symptoms.

Step 3: Consider to What Extent the Signs and Symptoms Are Related to Substances

The variety of substances that people use and misuse is remarkable, as are the clinical effects of substance use. Among older adults, alcohol, benzodiazepines, and nicotine are the most commonly used substances, so you should know the common effects of these substances (e.g., how the decrease in lean body mass and the decreased efficiency of alcohol metabolism among older adults prolong the effects of alcohol). However, these are not the only substances to consider. People can experience mental distress during substance use, intoxication, and withdrawal. When you seek the cause of a patient's distress, always consider drugs of abuse, as well as nonabused prescription, over-the-counter, and herbal medicines. Ask about substances ingested both intentionally and unintentionally, and remember that people often underreport their use of substances. Consider the following possibilities:

- The patient uses substances that directly cause her psychiatric signs and symptoms, as in a substance/medication-induced disorder.
- A patient uses substances because of a mental disorder and its sequelae.
- A patient uses substances and experiences psychiatric signs and symptoms, but the substance use and the signs and symptoms are unrelated.

Step 4: Consider to What Extent Signs and Symptoms Are Related to Another Medical Condition

A patient can present with another medical condition that mimics psychiatric signs and symptoms. This may be a sentinel event that occurs in advance of the other stigmata of a medical condition. Alternatively, a patient may develop psychiatric signs and symptoms years after presentation for another medical condition.

In caring for older adults, it is especially important to remember that persons change over time. You should be vigilant for the development of a neurocognitive or depressive disorder or an altered response to a previously well-tolerated medication following a stroke. In a hospital or other institutional setting, it is important to distinguish between enduring changes and temporary changes endemic to these settings, which are known to promote delirium. In general, clues that another medical condition may be related to a mental disorder include an atypical presentation, abnormal age at onset, and abnormal course. Consider these possibilities:

- Another medical condition directly alters psychiatric signs and symptoms.
- Another medical condition indirectly alters psychiatric signs and symptoms, such as through a psychological mechanism.
- The treatment for another medical condition directly alters psychiatric signs and symptoms.
- A mental disorder, or its treatment, causes or exacerbates another medical condition.
- A patient has both a mental disorder and another medical condition, but they are causally unrelated.

Step 5: Consider to What Extent the Signs and Symptoms Are Related to a Mental Disorder

DSM-5 diagnoses are summaries of information that allow you to categorize the experiences of a distressed person and to communicate with other professionals. You should rely on the predominant symptomatology to support your diagnosis. DSM-5 seeks parsimony, but diagnoses are not mutually exclusive, so consider these possibilities:

- Condition A predisposes a patient to Condition B and vice versa.
- An underlying condition, such as a genetic predisposition, may make a patient susceptible to both Conditions A and B.
- A mediating factor, such as alterations in reward systems, may influence susceptibility to both Conditions A and B.
- Conditions A and B may be part of a more complex and unified syndrome that has been artificially split in the diagnostic system.
- The relationship between Conditions A and B may be artificially enhanced by overlaps in the diagnostic criteria.
- The comorbidity between Conditions A and B may be coincidental.

Step 6: Consider Whether No Mental Disorder Is Present

"Normality" covers a wide range of behaviors and thoughts that vary across cultural groups and developmental stages. In DSM-5, a mental disorder causes a "clinically significant disturbance in an individual's cognition, emotion regulation, or behavior that reflects a dysfunction in the psychological, biological, or developmental processes underlying mental functioning" (American Psychiatric Association 2013, p. 20). When a patient's symptoms and presentation do not fulfill the criteria for a specific mental disorder but cause clinically significant distress or impairment, consider these alternatives:

- Other specified diagnosis—The practitioner specifies why a patient's experience does not meet the criteria of a specific diagnosis.
- Unspecified diagnosis—The practitioner does not specify why a patient's experience does not meet the criteria of a specific diagnosis.
- No psychiatric diagnosis at all—Many people live with one, two, or even more signs or symptoms of mental illness without meeting criteria for any DSM-5 mental disorder. After all, the boundaries between normality and abnormality are ultimately determined through the exercise of experienced judgment and increasing knowledge of the people you meet with the patients.

CHAPTER 10

The Mental Status Examination

A Psychiatric Glossary

JUST as a physical examination commonly moves from head to toe, the mental status examination begins with an older adult's outer appearance and progressively proceeds to his interior experiences. To describe these experiences, clinicians use a specialized language. Comprehensive glossaries of psychiatric terms are available elsewhere (e.g., Shahrokh et al. 2011). The following lists include brief definitions of some common specialized terms and serve as a format for organizing your findings in the mental status examination.

Appearance

Note the following about a person's appearance:

- Dress
- Cleanliness
- Habitus
- Posture
- Appropriateness for his age
- Ability to make and maintain eye contact

Behavior

Describe the patient's behaviors, including the following:

- Mannerisms (unnecessary behaviors that are a part of goal-directed behavior)

- Stereotypies (non-goal-directed behaviors)
- Drooling
- Tics (involuntary, recurrent, nonrhythmic movement or vocalization)
- Posturing (striking a pose and maintaining it)
- Presence of waxy flexibility (resistance of limbs to passive motion)
- Catalepsy (maintaining of any position)
- Tremor
- Agitation
- Movement retardation
- Akathisia (sense of restlessness accompanied by fidgeting, pacing, or being unable to stop moving)
- Signs of extrapyramidal symptoms or tardive dyskinesia
- Ambulatory status and, if possible, gait
- Ability to relate socially during your encounter

Speech

Describe the following characteristics of the patient's speech:

- Rate
- Tone
- Rhythm
- Volume
- General quality
- Presence of any latency (a pause of several seconds before responding to a question)

Document the following speech problems, if any:

- Anomia (inability to name everyday objects)
- Dysnomia (inability to find words)

Emotion

Older adults typically exhibit a more constricted emotional range than younger people. Document the following characteristics that contribute to a full description of an elder's emotional state:

- Quality
- Type

- Stability
- Range
- Intensity
- Appropriateness
- Mood (the emotional state that is sustained throughout your encounter)
- Affect (the often-fluctuating emotional tone that accompanies a person's speech and behaviors)
- Presence or absence of alexithymia (inability to describe or recognize one's own emotions)

Thought Process

Describe how a person thinks, and note any evidence of the following:

- Loosening of associations, which may be intact, circumstantial (patient provides unnecessary details but eventually answers a question), tangential (patient only touches on your question before heading in a different direction), or loose (patient's responses are unrelated to a question)
- Flight of ideas (an illogical group of associations)
- Word salad (random use of words)
- Distractibility (being easily diverted by extraneous stimuli)
- Derailment (running ideas into each other)
- Perseveration
- Verbigeration (prolonged repetition of isolated words)
- Echolalia (repetition of words or statements of others)
- Neologisms (creation of words)
- Clang association (words chosen purely for sound)
- Alliteration
- Pressured speech (increased, rapid speech that is often loud and difficult to interrupt)
- Decreased latency of response (answering of questions before you can finish asking them)
- Increased latency of response
- Poverty of speech
- Blocking (sudden stops in the middle of a thought sequence)
- Mutism (absence of speech)
- Aphonia (ability to only whisper or croak)

Thought Content

Comment on what a person discusses, including the presence of any of the following:

- Ideation, intent, or plan to harm self or others
- Phobia (intense, unreasonable fear)
- Obsession (idea, image, or desire that dominates thought)
- Compulsion (irresistible impulse to perform a behavior)
- Hallucination (perception of an absent stimulus)
- Illusion (misperception of an actual stimulus)
- Delusion (fixed, firm, false belief that is not part of a person's culture or religion)
- Persecution
- Paranoia
- Guilt
- Passivity
- Ideas of reference (perceptions that unrelated stimuli refer directly to the person)

Cognition and Intellectual Resources

Observe and comment on the patient's cognition and intellectual resources, including the following:

- Orientation
- Recent and remote memory
- Ability to calculate
- Ability to abstract and interpret proverbs

Insight/Judgment

Comment on the patient's insight and judgment, including the following:

- Insight into his condition, especially if he denies or appreciates his problems
- Judgment (the mental ability to compare choices and make decisions) as related to both presenting condition and age
- General appropriateness

CHAPTER 11

Selected DSM-5
Assessment Measures

DESPITE the popular perception that the DSM texts are chiseled in stone, the authors of DSM-5 (American Psychiatric Association 2013) describe the manual as subject to constant revision and have plans to update it in response to growing scientific knowledge. This commitment reaffirms that DSM is a pragmatic text for current clinical use (Kinghorn 2011). DSM-5's pragmatism extends to the authors' planning for its eventual successors. In DSM-5 Section III, "Emerging Measures and Models," the authors include several assessment tools, rating scales, and alternative diagnoses. Taken together, these constitute both valuable tools for current use and possible ways forward for DSM as a diagnostic system.

Currently, the main text of DSM-5 preserves the categorical model of mental illness. In this model, a person must meet certain criteria to have a mental illness on the basis of the presence or absence of symptoms. The categorical model was first introduced in DSM-III (American Psychiatric Association 1980) and is widely recognized for its improved diagnostic reliability, or in other words, the likelihood of different practitioners agreeing on the same diagnosis for a particular person. One shortcoming of this model is limited diagnostic validity—that is, the ability of practitioners to make an accurate diagnosis (Kendell and Jablensky 2003).

Each of the tools in Section III of DSM-5 attempts to improve the reliability and validity of psychiatric diagnoses. These tools are diverse, and we find that each one provides ways for practitioners to personalize the diagnostic criteria for particular patients.

In this chapter, we introduce several of these measures that can be useful in clinical practice with older adults.

Level 1 and Level 2 Cross-Cutting Symptom Measures

Most people first seek help for mental distress from someone they already know, often a primary care physician, clinic nurse, home health aide, or other practitioner whose training is outside mental health. In fact, most mental health care occurs outside the offices of mental health practitioners. To address the gap between the mental health training of non–mental health practitioners and the volume of mental health care they provide, DSM-5 offers screening tools—the Level 1 and Level 2 Cross-Cutting Symptom Measures—for use in either primary care or mental health settings. These brief, easy-to-read, paper-based tools can be completed before a clinical encounter, either by the patient or by someone who knows her well. The tools, which are available in Section III of DSM-5 and online at https://www.psychiatry.org/dsm5, can be reproduced and used, without additional permission, for clinical and research evaluations.

Each of these tools has a series of questions about recent symptoms (e.g., the Level 1 Cross-Cutting Symptom Measure—Adult asks, "During the past two [2] weeks, how much [or how often] have you avoided situations that make you anxious?"). These screening questions assess core symptoms for the major diagnoses. For example, for each Level 1 symptom statement, a patient or her caregiver will assess how much this bothered the patient using a 5-point scale: none (0), slight (1), mild (2), moderate (3), or severe (4). Each tool is designed to be easily scored. If a patient reports a clinically significant problem in any domain, you should consider a more detailed assessment tool (e.g., one designed for assessing anxiety).

The initial assessment to use with older adults is the Level 1 Cross-Cutting Symptom Measure—Adult, which contains 23 questions to be completed by the person seeking assessment before an initial evaluation or by the caregiver of an older adult. For most, but not all, of the symptom domains screened for in the Level 1 tool, there are separate Level 2 Cross-Cutting Symptom Measures for specific areas of concern, including depression, anger, mania, anxiety, somatic symptoms, sleep disturbances, repetitive thoughts and behaviors, and substance use.

Level 1 and 2 assessments initially help a practitioner identify and characterize the presenting problems. After the initial assessment, they can be used to help measure treatment response and progress toward recovery. The authors of DSM-5 suggest using the Cross-Cutting Symptom Measures at the first evaluation of a patient, in part to establish her baseline, and then revisiting that assessment periodically to assess her progress. These measures assess dimensions rather than diagnoses, which means they are not designed to tell the degree of likelihood of identifying a specific diagnosis. Their strength is that they allow you to track different symptom domains (e.g., the depressive symptoms of a patient with schizophrenia in addition to her psychotic symptoms).

Systematic use of these cross-cutting assessments will alert you to significant changes in a patient's symptomatology and will provide measurable outcomes for treatment plans. They also may alert researchers to lacunae in the current diagnostic system.

For your convenience, the Level 1 tool appears in Figure 11–1. Practitioners using the Level 1 tool are encouraged to further explore all reports of problems with inattention, psychosis, substance use, and suicidal ideation or attempts, even those rated as 1 (slight). For the other domains, practitioners are encouraged to explore symptoms rated 2 (mild) or greater. The Level 2 measures are easily accessed online at https://www.psychiatry.org/psychiatrists/practice/dsm/dsm-5/online-assessment-measures.

Cultural Formulation Interview

Another way the authors of DSM-5 have attempted to improve the diagnostic system is by attending to the cultural specificity of mental distress and illness. Asking about a patient's and caregiver's cultural understanding of sickness and health is an efficient way to build a therapeutic alliance while gathering pertinent information (Lim 2015). In addition, performing a cultural assessment also personalizes the diagnosis, which increases its accuracy (Bäärnhielm and Scarpinati Rosso 2009). In Section III of DSM-5, "Cultural Formulation" (pp. 749–759), the authors discuss cultural syndromes, idioms of distress, and explanations of perceived causes.

Name: _____ Age: _____ Sex: [ ] Male [ ] Female Date: _____

If the measure is being completed by an informant, what is your relationship with the individual?: _____

In a typical week, approximately how much time do you spend with the individual? _____ hours/week

Instructions: The questions below ask about things that might have bothered you. For each question, circle the number that best describes how much (or how often) you have been bothered by each problem during the past TWO (2) WEEKS.

		During the past TWO (2) WEEKS, how much (or how often) have you been bothered by the following problems?	None Not at all	Slight Rare, less than a day or two	Mild Several days	Moderate More than half the days	Severe Nearly every day	Highest Domain Score (clinician)
I.	1.	Little interest or pleasure in doing things?	0	1	2	3	4	
	2.	Feeling down, depressed, or hopeless?	0	1	2	3	4	
II.	3.	Feeling more irritated, grouchy, angry than usual?	0	1	2	3	4	
III.	4.	Sleeping less than usual, but still have a lot of energy?	0	1	2	3	4	
	5.	Starting lots more projects than usual or doing more risky things than usual?	0	1	2	3	4	
IV.	6.	Feeling nervous, anxious, frightened, worried, or on edge?	0	1	2	3	4	
	7.	Feeling panic or being frightened?	0	1	2	3	4	
	8.	Avoiding situations that make you anxious?	0	1	2	3	4	
V.	9.	Unexplained aches and pains (e.g., head, back, joints, abdomen, legs)?	0	1	2	3	4	
	10.	Feeling that your illnesses are not being taken seriously enough?	0	1	2	3	4	

FIGURE 11–1. DSM-5 Self-Rated Level 1 Cross-Cutting Symptom Measure—Adult

			0	1	2	3	4	
VI.	11.	Thoughts of actually hurting yourself?	0	1	2	3	4	
VII.	12.	Hearing things other people couldn't hear, such as voices even when no one was around?	0	1	2	3	4	
	13.	Feeling that someone could hear your thoughts, or that you could hear what another person was thinking?	0	1	2	3	4	
VIII.	14.	Problems with sleep that affected your sleep quality over all?	0	1	2	3	4	
IX.	15.	Problems with memory (e.g., learning new information) or with location (e.g., finding your way home)?	0	1	2	3	4	
X.	16.	Unpleasant thoughts, urges, or images that repeatedly enter your mind?	0	1	2	3	4	
	17.	Feeling driven to perform certain behaviors or mental acts over and over again?	0	1	2	3	4	
XI.	18.	Feeling detached or distant from yourself, your body, your physical surroundings, or your memories?	0	1	2	3	4	
XII.	19.	Not knowing who you really are or what you want out of life?	0	1	2	3	4	
	20.	Not feeling close to other people or enjoying your relationships with them?	0	1	2	3	4	

FIGURE 11–1. DSM-5 Self-Rated Level 1 Cross-Cutting Symptom Measure—Adult *(continued)*

		None Not at all	Slight Rare, less than a day or two	Mild Several days	Moderate More than half the days	Severe Nearly every day	Highest Domain Score (clinician)
	During the past **TWO (2) WEEKS**, how much (or how often) have you been bothered by the following problems?						
XIII.							
21.	Drink at least 4 drinks of any kind of alcohol in a single day?	0	1	2	3	4	
22.	Smoke any cigarettes, a cigar, or pipe, or use snuff or chewing tobacco?	0	1	2	3	4	
23.	Use any of the following medicines ON YOUR OWN, that is, without a doctor's prescription, in greater amounts or longer than prescribed [e.g., painkillers (like Vicodin), stimulants (like Ritalin or Adderall), sedatives or tranquilizers (like sleeping pills or Valium), or drugs like marijuana, cocaine or crack, club drugs (like ecstasy), hallucinogens (like LSD), heroin, inhalants or solvents (like glue), or methamphetamine (like speed)]?	0	1	2	3	4	

FIGURE 11–1. DSM-5 Self-Rated Level 1 Cross-Cutting Symptom Measure—Adult *(continued)*

Before we discuss using this cultural information in an interview, we should first define a few terms. A *cultural syndrome* is a group of clustered psychiatric symptoms specific to a particular culture or community. The syndrome may or may not be recognized as an illness by members of a community or by observers. A classic example is *ataque de nervios*, a syndrome of mental distress characterized by the sudden onset of intense fear, often experienced physically as a sensation of heat rising in the chest, that may result in aggressive or suicidal behavior (Lewis-Fernández et al. 2015). The syndrome is often associated with familial distress in Latino communities (Lizardi et al. 2009). A *cultural idiom of distress*, such as *ataque de nervios*, is a way of discussing mental distress or suffering shared by members of a particular community. Finally, a *cultural explanation* or *perceived cause* provides an explanatory model of why mental distress or illness occurs (American Psychiatric Association 2013). By its authors' own admission, DSM-5 is one culturally shaped way of accounting for distress; the authors state, "The current formulation acknowledges that *all* forms of distress are locally shaped, including the DSM-5 disorders" (American Psychiatric Association 2013, p. 758). So how do you acknowledge the effects of culture on distress?

The Cultural Formulation Interview (CFI) is a structured tool, updated for DSM-5, to assess the influence of culture in a particular patient's experience of distress. You can use the CFI at any time during an interview, but the authors of DSM-5 suggest using it when a patient seems disengaged, when you are struggling to reach a diagnosis, or when you are laboring to assess the dimensional severity of a diagnosis. Although use of the CFI has been studied mostly in immigrant communities (Martínez 2009), you should not limit its use to situations in which you perceive the patient as culturally different from yourself. You can use the CFI profitably in any setting because "cultural" accounts of why people get ill and why they return to health occur not only in immigrant communities but in all communities. Even when you believe that a person shares your own cultural account of illness and health, she may have a very different understanding of why people become ill and how they can become well. Furthermore, the CFI is the most patient-centered portion of DSM-5, and using it particularizes the diagnostic process.

The CFI is not a scored system of symptoms but rather a series of prompts to help you assess how a patient understands her distress, its etiology, its treatment, and the prognosis. The CFI can be incorporated into a diagnostic examination to personalize the diagnosis and build a therapeutic alliance. If you want to learn more about the CFI, you should review the materials in Section III of DSM-5 or read the *DSM-5 Handbook on the Cultural Formulation Interview* (Lewis-Fernández et al. 2015). The following is as an operationalized adaptation divided into five themes. Just as in the rest of this book, the italicized portions are interview prompts.

Introduction: *I would like to understand the problems that bring you here so that I can help you more effectively. I want to know about your experience and ideas. I will ask some questions about what is going on and how you are dealing with it. There are no right or wrong answers. I just want to know your views and those of other important people in your life.*

Cultural definition of the problem: *What problems or concerns bring you to the clinic? What troubles you most about your problem? People often understand their problems in their own way, which may be similar to or different from how doctors explain the problem. How would you describe your problem to someone else? Sometimes people use particular words or phrases to talk about their problems. Is there a specific term or expression that describes yours? If yes: What is it?*

Cultural perceptions of cause, context, and support: *Why do you think this is happening to you? What do you think are the particular causes of your problem? Some people may explain their problem as the result of bad things that happen in their life, problems with others, a physical illness, a spiritual reason, or some other cause. Do you? What, if anything, makes your problem worse, or makes it harder to cope with? What have your family, friends, and other people in your life done that may have made your problem worse? What, if anything, makes your problem better or helps you cope with it more easily?*

Role of cultural identity: *Is there anything about your background—for example, your culture, race, ethnicity, religion, or geographical origin—that is causing problems for you in your current life situation? If yes: In what way? On the other hand, is there anything about your background that helps you to cope with your current life situation? If yes: In what way?*

Cultural factors affecting self-coping and past help seeking: *Sometimes people have various ways to make themselves feel better. What have you done on your own to cope with your problem? Often, people also look for help from other individuals, groups, or institutions to help them feel better. In* the past, what kind of treatment or help from other sources have you sought for your problem? What type of help or treatment was most useful? How? What type of help or treatment was not useful? How? Has anything prevented you from getting the help you need—for example, cost or lack of insurance coverage, getting time off work or family responsibilities, concern about stigma or discrimination, or lack of services that understand your language or culture? If yes: What got in the way?

Cultural factors affecting current help seeking: *Now let's talk about the help you would be getting here from specialists in mental health. Is there anything about my own background that might make it difficult for me to understand or help you with your problem? How can I and others at our facility be most helpful for you? What kind of help would you like from us now?*

Conclusion: Thank the person for participation, summarize the main findings, and transition back to the remainder of your interview.

World Health Organization Disability Assessment Schedule 2.0

As part of their efforts to synchronize DSM with international diagnostic tools, the authors of DSM-5 have adopted the World Health Organization Disability Assessment Schedule 2.0 (WHODAS 2.0) to assess function in the following domains: cognition, mobility, self-care, getting along, life activities (household and school/work), and participation in society. WHODAS 2.0 is available in several versions: 12- and 36-question versions that can be self-administered, proxy administered, or interviewer administered (World Health Organization 2010).

DSM-5 includes the 36-item self-administered version of WHODAS 2.0 in Section III. You can learn more about WHODAS 2.0, learn how to interpret it, and find scoring sheets online at http://www.who.int/classifications/icf/whodasii/en.

Level of Personality Functioning Scale

The Alternative DSM-5 Model for Personality Disorders, presented in DSM-5 Section III, "Emerging Measures and Models," is used to consider a patient's personality traits in relation to her ability to function both personally and interpersonally. The Level of Personality Functioning Scale, reproduced below as Table 11–1, is included in DSM-5 to aid in this assessment. The interviewer is responsible for gathering sufficient clinical and historical information to differentiate five levels of functioning impairment, ranging from little or no impairment (Level 0) to extreme impairment (Level 4). The results of this evaluation can guide treatment planning and influence prognosis. However, given limited studies about personality disorders in older adults, findings should be interpreted with caution.

TABLE 11–1. Level of Personality Functioning Scale

Level of impairment	SELF		INTERPERSONAL	
	Identity	Self-direction	Empathy	Intimacy
0—Little or no impairment	Has ongoing awareness of a unique self; maintains role-appropriate boundaries. Has consistent and self-regulated positive self-esteem, with accurate self-appraisal. Is capable of experiencing, tolerating, and regulating a full range of emotions.	Sets and aspires to reasonable goals based on a realistic assessment of personal capacities. Utilizes appropriate standards of behavior, attaining fulfillment in multiple realms. Can reflect on, and make constructive meaning of, internal experience.	Is capable of accurately understanding others' experiences and motivations in most situations. Comprehends and appreciates others' perspectives, even if disagreeing. Is aware of the effect of own actions on others.	Maintains multiple satisfying and enduring relationships in personal and community life. Desires and engages in a number of caring, close, and reciprocal relationships. Strives for cooperation and mutual benefit and flexibly responds to a range of others' ideas, emotions, and behaviors.

TABLE 11–1. Level of Personality Functioning Scale *(continued)*

Level of impairment	SELF		INTERPERSONAL	
	Identity	Self-direction	Empathy	Intimacy
1—Some impairment	Has relatively intact sense of self, with some decrease in clarity of boundaries when strong emotions and mental distress are experienced. Self-esteem diminished at times, with overly critical or somewhat distorted self-appraisal. Strong emotions may be distressing, associated with a restriction in range of emotional experience.	Is excessively goal-directed, somewhat goal-inhibited, or conflicted about goals. May have an unrealistic or socially inappropriate set of personal standards, limiting some aspects of fulfillment. Is able to reflect on internal experiences, but may overemphasize a single (e.g., intellectual, emotional) type of self-knowledge.	Is somewhat compromised in ability to appreciate and understand others' experiences; may tend to see others as having unreasonable expectations or a wish for control. Although capable of considering and understanding different perspectives, resists doing so. Has inconsistent awareness of effect of own behavior on others.	Is able to establish enduring relationships in personal and community life, with some limitations on degree of depth and satisfaction. Is capable of forming and desires to form intimate and reciprocal relationships, but may be inhibited in meaningful expression and sometimes constrained if intense emotions or conflicts arise. Cooperation may be inhibited by unrealistic standards; somewhat limited in ability to respect or respond to others' ideas, emotions, and behaviors.

TABLE 11–1. Level of Personality Functioning Scale (*continued*)

| Level of impairment | SELF | | INTERPERSONAL | |
	Identity	Self-direction	Empathy	Intimacy
2—Moderate impairment	Depends excessively on others for identity definition, with compromised boundary delineation. Has vulnerable self-esteem controlled by exaggerated concern about external evaluation, with a wish for approval. Has sense of incompleteness or inferiority, with compensatory inflated, or deflated, self-appraisal. Emotional regulation depends on positive external appraisal. Threats to self-esteem may engender strong emotions such as rage or shame.	Goals are more often a means of gaining external approval than self-generated, and thus may lack coherence and/or stability. Personal standards may be unreasonably high (e.g., a need to be special or please others) or low (e.g., not consonant with prevailing social values). Fulfillment is compromised by a sense of lack of authenticity. Has impaired capacity to reflect on internal experience.	Is hyperattuned to the experience of others, but only with respect to perceived relevance to self. Is excessively self-referential; significantly compromised ability to appreciate and understand others' experiences and to consider alternative perspectives. Is generally unaware of or unconcerned about effect of own behavior on others, or unrealistic appraisal of own effect.	Is capable of forming and desires to form relationships in personal and community life, but connections may be largely superficial. Intimate relationships are predominantly based on meeting self-regulatory and self-esteem needs, with an unrealistic expectation of being perfectly understood by others. Tends not to view relationships in reciprocal terms, and cooperates predominantly for personal gain.

TABLE 11–1. Level of Personality Functioning Scale *(continued)*

Level of impairment	SELF		INTERPERSONAL	
	Identity	Self-direction	Empathy	Intimacy
3—Severe impairment	Has a weak sense of autonomy/agency; experience of a lack of identity, or emptiness. Boundary definition is poor or rigid: may show overidentification with others, overemphasis on independence from others, or vacillation between these. Fragile self-esteem is easily influenced by events, and self-image lacks coherence. Self-appraisal is un-nuanced: self-loathing, self-aggrandizing, or an illogical, unrealistic combination. Emotions may be rapidly shifting or a chronic, unwavering feeling of despair.	Has difficulty establishing and/or achieving personal goals. Internal standards for behavior are unclear or contradictory. Life is experienced as meaningless or dangerous. Has significantly compromised ability to reflect on and understand own mental processes.	Ability to consider and understand the thoughts, feelings, and behavior of other people is significantly limited; may discern very specific aspects of others' experience, particularly vulnerabilities and suffering. Is generally unable to consider alternative perspectives; highly threatened by differences of opinion or alternative viewpoints. Is confused about or unaware of impact of own actions on others; often bewildered about peoples' thoughts and actions, with destructive motivations frequently misattributed to others.	Has some desire to form relationships in community and personal life is present, but capacity for positive and enduring connections is significantly impaired. Relationships are based on a strong belief in the absolute need for the intimate other(s), and/or expectations of abandonment or abuse. Feelings about intimate involvement with others alternate between fear/rejection and desperate desire for connection. Little mutuality: others are conceptualized primarily in terms of how they affect the self (negatively or positively); cooperative efforts are often disrupted due to the perception of slights from others.

TABLE 11–1. Level of Personality Functioning Scale *(continued)*

| Level of impairment | SELF | | INTERPERSONAL | |
	Identity	Self-direction	Empathy	Intimacy
4—Extreme impairment	Experience of a unique self and sense of agency/autonomy are virtually absent, or are organized around perceived external persecution. Boundaries with others are confused or lacking. Has weak or distorted self-image easily threatened by interactions with others; significant distortions and confusion around self-appraisal. Emotions not congruent with context or internal experience. Hatred and aggression may be dominant affects, although they may be disavowed and attributed to others.	Has poor differentiation of thoughts from actions, so goal-setting ability is severely compromised, with unrealistic or incoherent goals. Internal standards for behavior are virtually lacking. Genuine fulfillment is virtually inconceivable. Is profoundly unable to constructively reflect on own experience. Personal motivations may be unrecognized and/or experienced as external to self.	Has pronounced inability to consider and understand others' experience and motivation. Attention to others' perspectives is virtually absent (attention is hypervigilant, focused on need fulfillment and harm avoidance). Social interactions can be confusing and disorienting.	Desire for affiliation is limited because of profound disinterest or expectation of harm. Engagement with others is detached, disorganized, or consistently negative. Relationships are conceptualized almost exclusively in terms of their ability to provide comfort or inflict pain and suffering. Social/interpersonal behavior is not reciprocal; rather, it seeks fulfillment of basic needs or escape from pain.

CHAPTER 12

Rating Scales and Alternative Diagnostic Systems

THERE are many ways to describe and measure distress. For example, a person may speak of having an *ataque de nervios*, whereas a practitioner may describe him as having a panic attack. Although the person and the practitioner may be describing the same experience, they are accounting for it in different ways. Typically, practitioners account for distress as a symptom of *disease*—that is, a pathological abnormality in the structure and function of body organs and systems—whereas patients account for distress as *illness*—that is, their personal experience of abnormality. Psychiatrists and other mental health practitioners currently account for mental distress as neither illness nor disease but rather as disorder. To name a collection of distressing symptoms as a disorder is an attempt to account for both pathological abnormalities and the effects of those abnormalities on a particular patient.

DSM-5 (American Psychiatric Association 2013) mental disorders are diagnostic labels rather than discrete biological phenomena. These diagnoses are provisional formulas for helping a person effect a change he could not make on his own. Within a particular diagnosis, there are very different experiences of symptoms and functional impairment. One older adult with panic attacks may need only to be taught breathing techniques, whereas another may need hospitalization and an extended course of therapy. One way to account for these differences in a patient's experience of a mental disorder is to use rating scales. Another is to use alternative diagnostic systems to describe the distress differently.

Rating Scales

Because we cannot yet diagnose and monitor most mental illnesses through physical means such as functional imaging, genetic testing, or blood serum tests, rating scales are important clinical aids to mental health care. Individual item responses on a standardized rating scale can be used to guide a clinical conversation (e.g., "You indicated that you sometimes have thoughts that you would be better off dead. Can you tell me more about that?"). Numerical scores on rating scales identify symptoms, guide diagnostic assessments, establish the severity of a disorder, and track the progress of patient care. Collecting these scale results over time will also enable measurement-based care, which refers to adjusting a patient's treatment plan until a measurable symptom target is reached.

We follow a few principles when considering how to use rating scales:

- Select scales that are research validated for age, condition, language, and (ideally) culture.
- Use broad-based screening scales to detect the likelihood of any disorder being present.
- Use a more specific rating scale to investigate a particular problem.
- Select brief rating scales to enhance patient cooperation and ease of implementation.
- Reserve longer rating scales for specialty settings.
- Remember that rating scales cannot make diagnoses—they are aids, not replacements, for clinician assessment.
- Recall that rating scale results depend on the reliability of the reporter and his interpretation.

There are hundreds of rating scales available; to assist your practice, we have listed in Table 12–1 the scales that we find especially helpful in the evaluation and care of older persons with mental distress. Many of these rating scales are (or can be) built into an electronic health record, which allows you to follow a patient's condition more objectively.

In addition, DSM-5 provides severity rating scales for many disorders. Most are specific to a particular disorder, and some include a narrative description to indicate that a particular disorder is mild, moderate, or severe. For some diagnoses, such as alcohol use disorder, severity depends on

TABLE 12–1. Select brief rating scales for use with older adults

Scale (common abbreviation)	Indication	Number of items	Reference/URL
Neurocognitive disorders			
Clock Drawing Test (CDT)	Assesses executive and visuospatial function	1	Shulman 2000
Confusion Assessment Method (CAM)	Assesses presence of delirium	9	Inouye et al. 1990 http://www.hospitalelderlifeprogram.org/delirium-instruments/
Frontal Assessment Battery (FAB)	Detects executive dysfunction affecting cognition and motor behavior	6	Dubois et al. 2000
Neuropsychiatric Inventory (NPI)	Assesses dementia-related behavioral symptoms	10, 12	Cummings et al. 1994 http://npitest.net/about-npi.html
Depression			
Geriatric Depression Scale (GDS)	Self-reporting depression screen	30	Yesavage et al. 1982–1983 https://web.stanford.edu/~yesavage/GDS.html

TABLE 12–1. Select brief rating scales for use with older adults *(continued)*

Scale (common abbreviation)	Indication	Number of items	Reference/URL
Patient Health Questionnaire (PHQ-9)	Self-reporting depression screen	9	Kroenke et al. 2001 http://www.phqscreeners.com
Executive functioning			
Executive Interview (EXIT)	Assesses executive function	25	Royall et al. 1992
Quick Executive Interview (Quick EXIT)	Assesses executive function	14	Larson and Heinemann 2010
Global mental status			
Mini-Mental State Examination (MMSE)	Assesses cognitive function and screens for dementia	30	Folstein et al. 1975
Montreal Cognitive Assessment (MoCA)	Detects mild cognitive impairment	30	Nasreddine et al. 2005 http://www.mocatest.org
Psychotic disorders			
Brief Psychiatric Rating Scale (BPRS)	Assesses presence and severity of psychotic symptoms	18	Overall and Gorham 1962

TABLE 12–1. Select brief rating scales for use with older adults *(continued)*

Scale (common abbreviation)	Indication	Number of items	Reference/URL
Substance use			
Alcohol-Related Problems Survey (ARPS)	Assesses alcohol use	20	Fink et al. 2002
Alcohol Use Disorders Identification Test (AUDIT)	Identifies problematic alcohol use	10	Babor et al. 1989 https://www.drugabuse.gov/sites/default/files/files/AUDIT.pdf
Short Michigan Alcoholism Screening Test—Geriatric Version (SMAST-G)	Screens for and detects problematic alcohol use	10	Blow et al. 1992

the number of criteria endorsed by a patient. For other diagnoses, such as a neurocognitive disorder, severity is measured by the degree to which a patient requires support. When appropriate, the severity ratings refer to specific measurements external to the mental status examination. For example, grading the severity of central sleep apnea depends, in part, on the extent of associated oxygen desaturation.

Alternative Diagnostic Systems

Although DSM-5 has been widely adopted, it is not the only way practitioners can describe and account for mental distress and mental illness. In different cultural and clinical situations, the diagnostic systems discussed in the following sections are in use.

INTERNATIONAL CLASSIFICATION OF DISEASES

The World Health Organization maintains its own diagnostic system, the International Classification of Diseases, commonly known by the abbreviation ICD. The clinical modification of the current, tenth revision (ICD-10-CM) includes mental disorders among a catalog of all medical diseases. The eleventh edition is under development and is due for release in 2017. Although most clinicians outside the United States use ICD-10 to diagnose mental disorders, it is less psychiatrically detailed than DSM-5 and was designed primarily to help epidemiologists track the incidence and prevalence of disease. DSM-5 includes ICD-10-CM codes, the U.S. clinical modification of the World Health Organization's ICD-10 codes. The World Health Organization authorized this adaption of ICD-10 for use in the United States. The ICD-10-CM codes found in DSM-5 are the only eligible codes for insurance reimbursement in the United States. The U.S. Centers for Medicare & Medicaid Services periodically updates ICD-10-CM codes to enhance their specificity to DSM-5 diagnoses. Any updates to ICD-10-CM codes after publication of DSM-5 can be found in the free DSM-5 Update at www.psychiatryonline.org.

RESEARCH DOMAIN CRITERIA

In 2010, the National Institute of Mental Health announced its intention to produce its own diagnostic system, the Research Domain Criteria (RDoC), in an attempt to unite symptoms with their underlying causes (Insel et al. 2010). At present, RDoC serves as an experimental framework for researching the biological origin of psychiatric illness. Rather than relying on the traditional clinical diagnostic system, this project has as its ultimate goal the mapping of behavioral patterns onto particular neural circuits, cells, genes, or molecules for which new research and new treatments could be developed. In this way, a specific behavioral pattern such as impulsivity, which is a trait that may occur in many different current DSM-5 diagnoses, might be found through the RDoC to have a relatively unified underlying biological cause. You can follow the progress of the development of the RDoC at http://www.nimh.nih.gov/research-priorities/rdoc/index.shtml.

CULTURE-SPECIFIC DIAGNOSTIC SYSTEMS

Several culture-specific psychiatric diagnostic systems are used in particular communities, including in Latin America (Berganza et al. 2002), Cuba (Otero-Ojeda 2002), China (Chen 2002), and Japan (Nakane and Nakane 2002). Anyone interested in the interface between DSM-5 and cultural psychiatry should read more about the Cultural Formulation Interview (Lewis-Fernández et al. 2015).

ICD-10-CM Z CODES

The authors of DSM-5 recommend the use of ICD-10-CM Z codes as a way to account for the psychosocial factors that are currently affecting a person's mental health and treatment. In Table 12–2, we include a truncated list of Z codes commonly used in elder mental health. ICD-10-CM Z codes are discussed further in Chapter 18, "Mental Health Treatment Planning."

TABLE 12–2. ICD-10-CM Z codes commonly used in elder mental health

ICD-10-CM Code	Description
Z00.4	General psychiatric examination, not elsewhere classified Exclusion: examination requested for medicolegal reasons (Z04.6)
Z04.6	General psychiatric examination, requested by authority
Z20.1	Contact with and exposure to tuberculosis
Z20.2	Contact with and exposure to infections with a predominantly sexual mode of transmission
Z20.5	Contact with and exposure to viral hepatitis
Z20.6	Contact with and exposure to human immunodeficiency virus (HIV) Exclusion: asymptomatic HIV infection status (Z21)
Z21	Asymptomatic HIV infection status
Z22.3	Carrier of other specified bacterial diseases
Z22.4	Carrier of infections with a predominantly sexual mode of transmission
Z22.5	Carrier of viral hepatitis
Z50.2	Alcohol rehabilitation
Z50.3	Drug rehabilitation
Z50.4	Psychotherapy, not elsewhere classified
Z51.5	Palliative care
Z55.0	Illiteracy and low-level literacy
Z56.0	Unemployment, unspecified
Z56.1	Change of job
Z56.2	Threat of job loss
Z56.3	Stressful work schedule
Z56.4	Discord with boss and workmates
Z56.5	Uncongenial work
Z56.6	Other physical and mental strain related to work

ICD-10-CM Code	Description
Z57.0	Occupational exposure to noise
Z57.1	Occupational exposure to radiation
Z57.2	Occupational exposure to dust
Z57.3	Occupational exposure to other air contaminants
Z57.4	Occupational exposure to toxic agents in agriculture
Z57.5	Occupational exposure to toxic agents in other industries
Z57.6	Occupational exposure to extreme temperature
Z57.7	Occupational exposure to vibration
Z58.0	Exposure to noise
Z58.1	Exposure to air pollution Exclusion: tobacco smoke
Z58.2	Exposure to water pollution
Z58.3	Exposure to soil pollution
Z58.4	Exposure to radiation
Z58.5	Exposure to other pollution
Z58.7	Exposure to tobacco smoke Inclusion: passive smoking
Z59.0	Homelessness
Z59.1	Inadequate housing Inclusion: lack of heating, restriction of space, technical defects in home preventing adequate care, unsatisfactory surroundings
Z59.2	Discord with neighbors, lodgers, and landlord
Z59.3	Problems related to living in residential institution
Z59.4	Lack of adequate food
Z59.5	Extreme poverty

ICD-10-CM Code	Description
Z59.6	Low income
Z59.7	Insufficient social insurance and welfare support
Z59.8	Other problems related to housing and economic circumstances Inclusion: foreclosure on loan, isolated dwelling, problems with creditors
Z60.0	Problems of adjustment to life-cycle transitions Inclusion: adjustment to retirement, empty nest syndrome
Z60.2	Living alone
Z60.3	Acculturation difficulty
Z60.4	Social exclusion and rejection Exclusion: target of adverse discrimination such as for racial or religious reasons
Z60.5	Target of perceived adverse discrimination and persecution
Z62.810	Personal history of physical and sexual abuse in childhood
Z63.0	Problems in relationship with spouse or partner
Z63.1	Problems in relationship with parents and in-laws
Z63.2	Inadequate family support
Z63.3	Absence of family member
Z63.4	Disappearance and death of family member
Z63.5	Disruption of family by separation and divorce
Z63.6	Dependent relative needing care at home
Z63.8	High expressed emotional level within family

ICD-10-CM Code	Description
Z64.2	Seeking and accepting physical, nutritional, and chemical interventions known to be hazardous and harmful Exclusion: substance dependence
Z64.3	Seeking and accepting behavioral and psychological interventions known to be hazardous and harmful
Z64.4	Discord with counselors Inclusion: with probation officer, social worker
Z65.0	Conviction in civil and criminal proceedings without imprisonment
Z65.1	Imprisonment and other incarceration
Z65.2	Problems related to release from prison
Z65.3	Problems related to other legal circumstances Inclusion: arrest, child custody or support proceedings, litigation, prosecution
Z65.4	Victim of crime and terrorism
Z65.5	Exposure to disaster, war, and other hostilities
Z70.0	Counseling related to sexual attitude
Z70.1	Counseling related to patient's sexual behavior and orientation
Z70.2	Counseling related to sexual behavior and orientation of third party
Z70.3	Counseling related to combined concerns regarding sexual attitude, behavior, and orientation
Z71.1	Person with feared complaint in whom no diagnosis is made
Z71.4	Alcohol abuse counseling and surveillance Exclusion: alcohol rehabilitation procedures
Z71.5	Drug abuse counseling and surveillance Exclusion: drug rehabilitation procedures

TABLE 12–2. ICD-10-CM Z codes commonly used in elder mental health *(continued)*

ICD-10-CM Code	Description
Z71.6	Tobacco abuse counseling Exclusion: tobacco rehabilitation procedures
Z72.0	Tobacco use Exclusion: tobacco dependence
Z72.1	Alcohol use Exclusion: alcohol dependence
Z72.2	Drug use Exclusion: abuse of non-dependence-producing substances, drug dependence
Z72.3	Lack of physical exercise
Z72.4	Inappropriate diet and eating habits
Z72.5	High-risk sexual behavior
Z72.6	Gambling and betting Exclusion: compulsive or pathological gambling
Z73.0	Burn-out
Z73.2	Lack of relaxation and leisure
Z73.6	Limitation of activities due to disability
Z74.0	Need for assistance due to reduced mobility
Z74.1	Need for assistance with personal care
Z74.2	Need for assistance at home and no other household member able to render care
Z74.3	Need for continuous supervision
Z75.0	Medical services not available in home
Z75.1	Person awaiting admission to adequate facility elsewhere
Z75.3	Unavailability and inaccessibility of health-care facilities
Z75.4	Unavailability and inaccessibility of other helping agencies
Z81.0	Family history of mental retardation
Z81.1	Family history of alcohol abuse
Z81.2	Family history of tobacco abuse

TABLE 12–2. ICD-10-CM Z codes commonly used in elder mental health *(continued)*

ICD-10-CM Code	Description
Z81.3	Family history of other psychoactive substance abuse
Z81.4	Family history of other substance abuse
Z81.8	Family history of other mental and behavioral disorders
Z91.1	Personal history of noncompliance with medical treatment and regimen
Z91.2	Personal history of poor personal hygiene
Z91.3	Personal history of unhealthy sleep-wake schedule
Z91.5	Personal history of self-harm Inclusion: parasuicide, self-poisoning, suicide attempt
Z91.6	Personal history of other physical trauma

Source. Buck 2017.

CHAPTER 13

Psychoeducational Interventions

Psychoeducation Classes

Elise is a 68-year-old woman who was diagnosed in her early 20s with bipolar I disorder, hypertension, and poorly controlled diabetes. She has responded well to a combination of valproic acid and sertraline. Over the past 40 years, however, her treatment course has been compromised because she intermittently stops medications when she is euthymic, resulting in hypomanic or depressive episodes and, occasionally, hospitalization for manic episodes. Elise does not understand the need to take medications when she is feeling well. Her daughter Mabel became involved last month when Elise was hospitalized for hyperosmolar hyperglycemic nonketotic syndrome. Elise once again had stopped her medications, become slightly paranoid during her hypomanic episode, and refused diabetes medications because she was convinced they were contaminated. She is now taking all her medications as recommended; however, you are concerned about the medical consequences if she stops again. Mabel explains that she became frustrated and estranged from her mother when Elise refused to take medications consistently and ended up in the hospital. You recommend that Mabel and Elise attend family-focused psychoeducation courses and join the local National Alliance on Mental Illness (NAMI) chapter.

Psychoeducation classes are a crucial but underemphasized part of mental health treatment that are typically recommended for patients with severe mental illnesses (e.g., schizophrenia, bipolar disorder, and major depressive disorder) and their identified caregivers. These classes provide information to both patients and caregivers about the disorders and what to expect from treatment. Because caregivers frequently administer medications or ensure compliance, help reinforce the treatment plan, and notify practitioners when they recognize early signs of patient relapse, their involvement is critical to the success of psychoeducation. The classes have several key components: education about mental health disorders, information about how to access acute and chronic care resources, skill training for the management of disorders, problem-solving skills, and support for caregivers (Substance Abuse and Mental Health Services Administration 2009). Another major theme is collaboration between practitioner, patient, and caregivers. Collaboration can be especially challenging because patients may have limited insight into their mental health disorder and no motivation to comply with their treatment plan; focusing on concrete goals such as staying out of the hospital can be more productive. Psychoeducation classes usually last 9–10 months and can be conducted with a single family or multiple families at the same time.

Most psychoeducation effectiveness studies focus on severe mental illness in the general adult population. Because older adults typically experience some degree of cognitive decline and are often prescribed more complex medication regimens than younger adults, it is necessary to customize psychoeducational interventions for them. Unfortunately, this customization occurs with limited evidence because, to date, few studies have addressed the effectiveness of psychoeducation among older adults, although available studies generally support it. For example, in a study by Sherrill et al. (1997), classes for older adults with recurrent major depressive disorder and their families were well received, and regular attendance was associated with a higher likelihood of patients remaining in treatment during the maintenance phase of depression. In a preliminary study by Depp et al. (2007), medication adherence skills training for older adults with bipolar disorder was also well received and was associated with improvement in adherence and management, depressive symptoms, and quality-of-life measures. In contrast to these studies, a randomized controlled trial comparing psychoeducation for patients with major neurocognitive disorder versus standard care did not show any differences in caregiver burden (Martín-Carrasco et al. 2014). Another psychoeducational intervention for caregivers of patients with major neurocognitive disorder, however, showed improved caregiver competence (Llanque et al. 2015). Additional studies are needed to develop evidence-based psychoeducation programs for older adults.

Nonpharmacological Interventions for Cognitive and Behavioral Difficulties

Over the next several months, you notice that Elise is having difficulty following some conversations, even though she insists that her mood is euthymic. You are concerned about medication compliance because she has episodes of hyperglycemia when she cannot remember to take insulin with meals. Mabel tells you that Elise is having cognitive difficulties with organizing complex tasks, such as knowing how to draw up and adjust the timing of her insulin, and cannot easily recall recent events. You refer Elise for a neuropsychological evaluation to determine whether she has a major neurocognitive disorder; the evaluation confirms your suspicion that she does have major neurocognitive disorder superimposed on bipolar disorder.

When you discuss this new diagnosis with Mabel, she complains that Elise is easily agitated, so you ask her to describe this agitation in more detail. Mabel explains that her mother sometimes resists insulin injections, yells or tries to walk away, and once almost stuck her with the needle. Mabel finds giving multiple injections quite frustrating and often does not even offer the long-acting insulin dose at night because she is so tired of trying to persuade Elise to agree. As you investigate this behavioral disturbance, you learn that Elise cannot consistently remember that she has diabetes, so you create a plan that will minimize her need for insulin injections and set a higher hemoglobin A_{1c} target goal because of her diagnosis of major neurocognitive disorder. You consult with your colleagues in geriatric medicine, endocrinology, and pharmacy to devise a diabetes medication regimen that requires only one injection of long-acting insulin per day and use of oral hypoglycemics.

Now when Mabel gives Elise an injection, she picks a time when Elise feels most relaxed and puts on music for distraction. She gives Elise a stuffed animal to hold so she is less likely to grab the hand holding the syringe. You advise Mabel to give Elise her regular evening trazodone about 30 minutes before the injection so she will be drowsy and more cooperative. The nutritionist works with Mabel to decrease Elise's insulin by ensuring that only diabetic-friendly foods are present in the household. Elise had been snacking on cookies and eating ice cream, which increased her insulin requirement. Finally, Mabel and Elise work with the occupational therapist to develop physical activities that should further decrease the need for insulin. When you evaluate the effectiveness of your plan after 3 months, you learn that Elise's episodes of agitation have resolved and the number of hyperglycemic episodes has decreased by 25% since she began consistently taking the long-acting insulin injection given once a day by her daughter.

The DICE (Describe, Investigate, Create, and Evaluate) model is a well-established multidisciplinary intervention for patients who have major neurocognitive disorder with behavioral disturbance; its purpose is to reduce the usage of psychotropic medications in these patients (Kales et al. 2014). In the Describe step, a caregiver tells the practitioner about the behavioral event in as much detail as possible. The practitioner should ask questions to learn whom this event occurs around (a certain family member, the new home health aide, or everyone), what exactly is happening (a step-by-step description or even a cell phone recording of the event can be helpful), when it happens (does it occur more frequently at night or during the day?), and where it takes place (in public or at home). In the Investigate step, the practitioner considers any symptoms of the neurocognitive disorder, medications, lifestyle habits (sleep, physical, and social activity), and caregiver factors (caregiver's physical health and social activity) that may result in the behavior. In the Create step, the practitioner develops a plan to address the behavioral disturbance. The plan should include modification of the patient's activity and environment plus education about and modification of the caregiver's approach. In the Evaluate step, the plan is assessed for effectiveness and to determine whether further modification is needed.

Many practitioners feel stuck when they create, evaluate, or modify plans that do not work. Often, these plans do not work because practitioners have been trained to develop only pharmacological interventions rather than nonpharmacological ones. Practitioners should recognize the importance of consulting other disciplines that specialize in nonpharmacological management of patients, including but not limited to geriatric medicine, rehabilitation (occupational, physical, and recreational therapy), pharmacy, and nursing. They should also consult their own colleagues to see if they have other ideas. For the practitioner who is willing to learn, there are many effective nonpharmacological interventions available (Alzheimer's Association 2015b; American Occupational Therapy Association 2016; Gitlin et al. 2012). As we saw in Elise's situation, initiating changes that improve the physical and mental health of an older adult often requires the participation of practitioners from several disciplines.

Support Groups

Because patients and their caregivers often experience mental illness as alienating, both benefit from understanding support networks. A practitioner can encourage joining a support group to help decrease any stigma and isolation that patients and caregivers may experience. We usually recommend that caregivers of patients with severe mental illness reach out to NAMI, whereas caregivers of patients with neurocognitive disorders should contact the Alzheimer's Association. Caregivers can also use Internet-based tools such as Link2Care (http://lists.caregiver.org/mailman/listinfo/link2care_ discussion_lists.caregiver.org) and the Comprehensive Health Enhancement Support System (www.chess.wisc.edu/chess/ home/home.aspx), especially if they are unable to leave the home because of their duties (Collins and Swartz 2011).

Mobile Apps and Web-Based Resources

MOBILE APPS

For tech-savvy older adults, mobile apps provide the ability to monitor, maintain, and improve mental health. PTSD Coach (available for free at https://mobile.va.gov) is one example of a mobile app that can be useful for providing "e-guidance" to patients with mental health disorders. MapMyWalk (available at http://www.mapmywalk.com) is an app that helps older adults visualize and increase their activity. Although apps are growing in popularity, evidence for their efficacy remains limited.

WEB RESOURCES FOR EDUCATING PATIENTS, CAREGIVERS, AND PRACTITIONERS

Because practitioners are busy and rarely have enough time to respond to all of their patients' questions about diagnoses and treatments, many patients and caregivers look online for answers. It is important that patients and caregivers access reliable Web sites so they do not make decisions that compromise their medical care, such as making incorrect self-diagnoses or discontinuing medications because of unwarranted fear of adverse effects. A reliable Web-based resource can provide information about issues such as suicide in a safe environment so patients and caregivers do not feel stigmatized. They may not know where to turn in a crisis and may feel overwhelmed by the difficulty of accessing mental health resources due to underinsurance or the lack of available mental health practitioners in their area. Practitioners should have on hand an up-to-date list of Web sites to give to the tech-savvy patient or caregiver. Below is a list of Web sites that can be useful.

- **Alzheimer's Association (http://www.alz.org)**. Patients with Alzheimer's disease and their caregivers will find a wealth of medical information, caregiver tips, and details about the financial and legal issues affecting patients and their families. The site also provides information about how to connect to local chapters and a 24/7 hotline for caregivers to call.
- **American Foundation for Suicide Prevention (https://afsp.org)**. Suicide is a difficult topic for patients, caregivers, and practitioners to discuss. This Web site provides resources for patients, concerned caregivers, and anyone who has lost a loved one to suicide. It also provides information about how to connect to local chapters and a 24/7 suicide hotline.
- **Association for Frontotemporal Degeneration (http://www.theaftd.org)**. Patients with early-onset, rapidly progressive dementias such as frontotemporal dementia have significantly different behavioral issues from patients with Alzheimer's disease and other more common types of dementia. Early onset of the dementia is often a devastating shock for caregivers and family members. This Web site provides information about early-onset dementias and other useful resources for this population's unique needs.

- **National Alliance on Mental Illness (http://www. nami.org)**. NAMI plays a major role in the support and education of family members and friends who have a loved one with a mental illness, whether diagnosed or undiagnosed. Information is available about various mental health disorders. Family members and friends often find it helpful to connect with their local chapters to find support groups. This organization is particularly helpful for patients who are diagnosed with severe mental illness such as bipolar disorder, schizophrenia, posttraumatic stress disorder, or depression.
- **National Institute of Mental Health (https://www.nimh. nih.gov)**. The National Institute of Mental Health is an invaluable resource for learning about mental health and the most up-to-date research. The health and education section provides information about mental health treatment that can be easily understood by a general audience. News about clinical trials can also be easily accessed here.
- **NIH Senior Health (http://nihseniorhealth.gov)**. This National Institutes of Health Web site provides excellent information for practitioners, patients, and caregivers. The emphasis on healthy lifestyle and health maintenance will appeal to older adults who do not have a mental health disorder but need to address lifestyle issues.
- **UpToDate (http://www.uptodate.com)**. This Web resource, available through many academic institutions and hospitals, is normally used by practitioners to learn about the latest recommendations for clinical treatment. Patient information is also available on a wide range of topics, including specific medications. Handouts are available for beginning and advanced levels of health literacy.

CHAPTER 14

Psychosocial Interventions

Stefan is a 92-year-old man with major neurocognitive disorder due to Alzheimer's disease, congestive heart failure with an ejection fraction of 20%, right hip fracture with a history of open reduction and internal fixation, hypertension, and chronic kidney disease stage 3 who presents with his daughter Rene. Rene, who had been working full time, became involved in her parents' care 3 months ago after Stefan's wife, Amélie, had a heart attack and was hospitalized for a week. Rene had to unexpectedly take time off from her job but now works part time from home so she can help care for Stefan and Amélie, who have moved into Rene's home. Rene has no assistance and feels overwhelmed caring for both of her parents.

You refer Rene to a social worker to consider various options to assist with care for her parents. They discuss case management, home health services, respite services, and the local Program of All-Inclusive Care for the Elderly (PACE). Rene decides to hire home health services 5 days a week for 12 hours. At her next visit, she reports decreased caregiver stress.

Determining What Services Patients Need

As the population ages, living options for older people are increasing. When patients and caregivers consider the choices, they may easily feel overwhelmed by the variety of terms whose meanings, except for *nursing homes* and *skilled nursing facilities*, are not regulated. Given the complexity of the options, practitioners should consider at least a one-time consultation with a social worker, case manager, or local aging agency. Before the practitioner consults with these people, he should first answer two important questions: 1) What is the patient's minimum required level of care (e.g., skilled nursing, help with medications and transportation)? 2) What private and public resources does the patient have that can be spent on his care? Which services are provided and which are not, as well as the payment mechanism, should be clarified in detail at every facility that is considered.

ASSESSING PATIENTS FOR SERVICE NEEDS

Assessing an older patient for his needs can seem complicated and overwhelming for the practitioner. To simplify this process, we recommend breaking down the assessment for service needs into three steps: 1) assess the patient's functional abilities and gait, 2) assess the patient's cognition and behavior, and 3) assess the patient's finances.

STEP 1: ASSESS FUNCTIONAL ABILITIES AND GAIT

The first step in determining what services a patient needs or where he can live is to understand his functional abilities. Formal, detailed functional assessment of activities of daily living (ADLs) may require a referral to occupational therapy. However, you also can use short clinician-administered assessments, some of which require caregiver or patient ratings. Several such assessments of ADLs are summarized in Table 14–1.

In addition to these functional assessments for older patients, it is critical to assess the patient's gait, which is a proxy for mobility and ability to function independently and often is an indication of physical and mental illness. The structured tools summarized in Table 14–2 can be used to assess an older adult's gait.

One-third of all older adults fall each year, and one-fifth of all falls result in a serious injury (Centers for Disease Control and Prevention 2016). Because falls are a significant source of morbidity and mortality among older adults, a practitioner must ally with a patient and his caregivers to prevent falls (Tinetti and Kumar 2010). One important way to reduce the risk of falls is to complete an environmental assessment of the places where an older adult lives and frequently visits. An environmental assessment will include both a "diagnosis"—including an assessment of a patient's footwear and an assessment of the structure of his dwelling (e.g., stairs, doorways, handrails, grab bars)—and a "prescription"—the removal of known obstacles (e.g., clutter, electrical cords, loose rugs), the provision of adequate foot-

TABLE 14–1. Assessments of activities of daily living

Scale	Indication	Rater	Number of items	Reference/URL
Barthel Index of Activities of Daily Living	Assesses mobility and ability to perform self-care	Patient or caregiver	10	Collin et al. 1988 https://www.healthcare.uiowa.edu/igec/tools/function/barthelADLs.pdf
Instrumental Activities of Daily Living	Measures complex functions correlated with independent functioning	Patient or caregiver	8	Lawton and Brody 1969 https://www.healthcare.uiowa.edu/igec/tools/function/lawtonbrody.pdf
Katz Index of Independence in Activities of Daily Living	Monitors ability to perform self-care	Caregiver or practitioner	6	Katz et al. 1963 https://clas.uiowa.edu/sites/clas.uiowa.edu.socialwork/files/NursingHomeResource/documents/Katz%20ADL_LawtonIADL.pdf
Palliative Performance Scale	Assesses and monitors physical and functional status of a person receiving palliative care	Practitioner	5	Anderson et al. 1996

TABLE 14–2. Assessments of gait, immobility, and fall risk

Scale	Indication	Rater	Number of items	Reference
Berg Balance Scale	Assesses balance and predicts fall risk	Practitioner	14	Berg et al. 1992
Get-up and Go Test	Assesses gait and balance	Practitioner	8-step movement	Mathias et al. 1986
Performance-Oriented Assessment of Balance	Assesses balance	Practitioner	13-step movement	Tinetti 1986
Performance-Oriented Assessment of Gait	Assesses gait	Practitioner	9-step movement	Tinetti 1986

wear, a review of a patient's medications, and, often, balance and gait training. Although occupational and physical therapists are often the community experts in these evaluations, several checklists have been designed for use by any practitioner. These assessments include the Gerontological Environmental Modifications Assessment (Bakker 2005) and the Check for Safety: A Home Fall Prevention Checklist for Older Adults (Centers for Disease Control and Prevention 2015).

STEP 2: ASSESS COGNITION AND BEHAVIOR

The second step to understanding where your patient can live is to make sure you have a thorough understanding of the patient's current and potential future problems with cognition and behavior. This is important because you have to be able to help caregivers plan for the future. For example, a pleasant patient with early Alzheimer's disease may not need a locked dementia unit immediately, but you should recommend that the caregivers focus on finding places that have locked units in their facilities. Then, in the event that the patient starts to wander, his caregiver can easily arrange for him to be moved to a locked unit without going through the placement process again.

The most comprehensive tests of cognitive and behavioral function are conducted by neuropsychologists. Neuropsychological testing for neurocognitive and psychiatric disorders usually includes a detailed clinical history based on information from the patient and caregiver, an objective assessment of the patient's functioning prior to the onset of the mental health disorder, and a battery of tests to understand which disorders are contributing to the patient's current clinical presentation. Neuropsychologists can carefully select tests on the basis of the clinical presentation and complaint, or they can use a fixed, comprehensive assessment. Neuropsychological testing is different from cognitive screens such as the Montreal Cognitive Assessment (MoCA) or the Mini-Mental State Examination (MMSE), which can be completed in only a few minutes. Neuropsychological testing may take anywhere from 2 to 6 hours. Neuropsychologists who have extensive experience working with older adults will generally keep the batteries on the shorter side or provide frequent breaks because they recognize that older adults will tire easily. Poor effort due to a patient's exhaustion is a common reason for invalid test results.

A common complaint of many practitioners is that neuro-psychology reports do not help them understand a patient with complex neurocognitive and psychiatric issues because the report comes back with "a laundry list of potential problems" that the practitioners already knew existed. The secret to getting back a report that helps you is to understand that neuropsychology testing is similar to a surgical operation. To increase the likelihood of a good outcome (i.e., getting a report that helps you), make sure you "prep" your patient by doing the following:

1. Refer older patients to neuropsychologists who are board certified or board eligible, and preferably who have geriatric experience, to ensure a high-quality, valid assessment. (This is similar to when you refer your patients to a board-certified surgeon who is well versed in a highly specialized procedure.)
2. Address all visual and hearing impairment problems beforehand because these can affect test performance.
3. Send all records, including test results of brain imaging, prior to the assessment to give the neuropsychologist ample time to review the records and determine additional appropriate tests. Because of the anatomic detail provided, magnetic resonance imaging is significantly preferable to computed tomography scans.
4. Do your best to effectively treat all psychiatric symptoms such as depression, mania, and psychosis.
5. Minimize or stop a patient's cognitively impairing medications, such as anticholinergics, benzodiazepines, and sedating pain medications, as well as excessive substance use, for at least 1 month prior to testing.
6. Most importantly, write a clear question or statement listing potential diagnoses that you think might contribute to the patient's problem. The following are not helpful referral questions: "Cognitive impairment?" and "Can this person drive or manage his finances independently?" A much better referral is something such as the following: "I am wondering whether my patient has major neurocognitive disorder, major depressive disorder, or bipolar disorder with depression. I am also concerned about his ability to safely drive and live alone." Because many neuropsychologists design a test battery on the basis of the referral question or statement, the better worded your re-

ferral, the better the neuropsychologist can design the battery of tests and address your concerns.

When you receive the neuropsychologist's report, do not feel overwhelmed by the jargon (e.g., "significant difficulties with executive function such as organization and planning"). Feel free to call the neuropsychologist about what the results mean in terms of the problems your patient is facing. Neuropsychologists are bona fide clinicians and will appreciate this call. Finally, these neuropsychology reports are invaluable for other specialists, particularly occupational therapists and geropsychologists. When you share these reports with these specialists, they can help you figure out what to do about the problems the neuropsychologist describes. For example, problems with organization and planning indicate that the patient is feeling overwhelmed by anything that requires multiple steps. Specialists may approach these problems in different ways. An occupational therapist may recommend using a checklist to complete a complex task as part of cognitive rehabilitation. A geropsychologist may decide to use problem-solving therapy so the patient feels less overwhelmed about how to solve a problem.

STEP 3: ASSESS FINANCES

The third step in determining where a patient can live is to arrange for a financial assessment by a social worker or case manager. Although social workers and case managers are tremendously helpful in figuring out which services patients qualify for, you can make the process go faster by having your patient and his caregivers collect all the paperwork about assets belonging to both the patient and the spouse (if there is one), including but not limited to bank accounts, retirement accounts, pensions, property, and any other sources of income. Patients should also locate basic identifying information documents, such as birth certificate and Social Security card, because they may need them when applying for Medicaid or completing social services applications. Bringing all of this paperwork to the first visit for a financial assessment will save your patient and his caregiver an extra visit.

CONSIDERING AT-HOME SERVICE OPTIONS

CASE MANAGEMENT

Case management is typically handled by a nurse or social worker who is responsible for coordinating and implementing a patient's care plan to improve management of his chronic illness. A review by the Agency for Healthcare Research and Quality found that case management for older adults with complex chronic medical illnesses at best had only a small impact on patient-centered outcomes, quality of care, and resource utilization; however, patients with complex medical illnesses did feel that their care was better coordinated, and caregivers reported less depression and stress (Hickam et al. 2013). Case management is a highly heterogeneous approach; the most successful interventions include longer contact time with clients, face-to-face meetings, and integration with practitioners.

Health insurance may cover case management under special circumstances, but many times patients and caregivers will need to pay out of pocket to hire a geriatric case manager. If they do hire someone privately, it must be a person with an active license in his area of expertise and experience working with older adults.

RESPITE PROGRAMS

Caregiving can be emotionally and physically exhausting. Because the judicious use of respite programs can prevent caregiver burnout, practitioners should discuss the availability of respite care early, instead of waiting until a caregiver burns out and the need for services becomes acute. The three major types of respite programs are home care services, adult day health centers, and brief stays at residential facilities. Home care services range from providing assistance with ADLs and light household chores to providing companionship. Adult day health centers offer supervised care for those who need medical and social services. Many of these centers provide transportation, meals, and some health-related services such as assistance with ADLs. Some also provide assistance for special populations, such as patients with dementia (National Adult Day Services Association 2016). Finally, certain residential facilities allow for brief stays ranging from a night, to a weekend, to a few weeks. Veterans who are eligible for VA medical care can receive respite services free of charge from the

VA (U.S. Department of Veterans Affairs 2016). Otherwise, Medicare and many forms of health insurance do not cover most types of respite services (Alzheimer's Association 2016).

PACE

PACE provide comprehensive medical and social services to frail adults age 55 and older who live in a PACE organization service area and have needs equivalent to those of persons currently in nursing homes (Medicaid.gov 2016a, 2016b). The purpose of PACE is to allow individuals who would normally enter a nursing home to stay at home instead. Most of the adults who are enrolled in PACE are dually eligible for Medicaid and Medicare; instead of the traditional fee-for-service model, capitation is used. Currently, there are more than 100 PACE programs in 32 states.

HOME HEALTH SERVICES

Home health services allow many older people to continue living at home, even as their physical need for care increases, rather than being placed in a long-term-care setting. The wide range of possible home health services includes occupational and physical therapy, speech therapy, skilled nursing, assistance with ADLs, assistance with cooking and light housekeeping, and medication monitoring. Patients and their caregivers are urged to investigate options with a social worker or case manager (http://www.eldercare.gov/eldercare.net/public/resources/factsheets/home_health_care.aspx).

LONG-TERM-CARE PLANNING

Stefan does well with home health services for about 2 years but then has a fall resulting in a hip fracture. He requires emergency surgery and becomes wheelchair bound. Rene asks to talk to the social worker again because she is unable to care for both Stefan and her mother at home. After lengthy discussion with the social worker, Rene decides that her father needs a skilled nursing facility and her mother needs to move to an assisted living facility.

No matter what a patient's age or degree of disability, caregivers should be prepared for the possibility that patients will move at least once in their postretirement life. Patients who have planned retirement to a sunny locale for their 60s–80s may realize when they reach their 90s that they need to be closer to family for support. Caregivers may then find that they must find another facility as the patient physically declines and requires a higher level of care. The following are places older people can go: retirement communities, assisted living facilities, skilled nursing facilities, and long-term-care facilities.

Long-term-care planning is an important but difficult topic to bring up with your patients. Ideally, the conversation should begin when a person still has the capacity to express his feelings about placement and can be engaged in a meaningful dialogue. The natural reaction of many patients when approached about their future, independent of current mental or functional status, is to want to stay home. They may feel uncomfortable thinking of themselves as being sick enough to depend on others, especially in an institutionalized setting. Therefore, it is fairly common for the discussion about placement in a higher level of care to begin when patients are already in the hospital with significant functional decline and are unable to participate in decision making. Practitioners should provide information about long-term-care planning before meeting for a discussion so that patients and caregivers can come prepared with questions and concerns (http://longtermcare.gov/the-basics/what-is-long-term-care/).

Even when it is beyond the physical and/or mental capacity of their loved ones, caregivers often feel obligated to keep their loved ones at home for various reasons. Extending the caregiver network can sometimes allow the patient to stay home longer, but this is not always possible. Even the most dedicated caregiver may feel like a failure when watching a loved one move to a higher-level care facility. Also, such a move does not necessarily reduce the stress of caregivers, who often spend many hours visiting their loved ones, making sure they are properly cared for by the staff, and going to numerous medical visits.

Eldercare.gov provides a brochure to help patients and caregivers understand their housing options (http://www.eldercare.gov/eldercare.net/public/Resources/Brochures/docs/Housing_Options_Booklet.pdf). For patients who are fairly independent with instrumental activities of daily living (IADLs) and may need only more structured socialization, prepared meals, and light household assistance, independent living or retirement communities may be a good fit. For those who require assistance with IADLs (such as medication management) and some help with ADLs but do not have an identified skilled nursing need, assisted living facilities may be a good fit (http://www.eldercare.gov/eldercare.net/public/resources/factsheets/assisted_living.aspx). Finally, long-term-care and skilled nursing facilities require patients to have at least one documented skilled nursing need. Skilled nursing facilities are expensive, and Medicaid is the primary payer for about 63% of these residents (Harrington et al. 2015).

FINANCIAL PLANNING

Only a small number of patients can afford to pay for long-term care or have purchased long-term-care insurance (Feder and Komisar 2012). For most patients and their families, paying for long-term care is an expensive proposition. If possible, financial planning care should occur well before it is needed. Financial advisers who have experience with long-term-care planning for older adults can be quite helpful. It is often a good idea for the patient to appoint someone who will make decisions when the patient can no longer do so because of significant illness. It is simpler to choose one person to be in charge of both finances and health care; however, if two different people are appointed, ideally, they should share a similar vision about the patient's care.

Covering the cost of long-term care and other services will vary widely on the basis of the patient's access to public and private resources. Information on how to pay for these services is available online (http://longtermcare.gov/costs-how-to-pay/).

When a patient no longer has the capacity to sign paperwork to designate a decision maker or when there is familial discord, consultation with an eldercare attorney may be necessary to determine whether guardianship proceedings (often an expensive process) will be necessary.

ADVANCE DIRECTIVE PLANNING

Advance directive planning is an important element of a patient's long-term-care plan and should be included in any discussion of treatment goals, life expectancy, and long-term care. Despite universal recommendations for advance directives, they are often not completed even by those who are older and medically frail (Benson and Aldrich 2012). Less than one-third of home health care patients and less than three-fourths of nursing home residents have an advance directive on record (Jones et al. 2011). Advance care planning can reduce expensive and unwanted treatments for older adults. Without advance directives, physicians frequently err on the side of overtreatment (Billings 2012). A notable statistic is that about 5% of Medicare beneficiaries who die use about 25% of overall Medicare spending in the last year of their life (Austin and Fleisher 2003; Hogan et al. 2001).

Nevertheless, many practitioners are reluctant to discuss advance directives because they fear the discussions will be time-consuming. Only 65%–76% of physicians of patients who did complete an advance directive were aware of its existence (Kass-Bartelmes 2003). The clinical key is to introduce the idea at the end of a visit, give the patient and his caregiver information about advance directives, and continue the conversation at the next encounter. Advance directives do not involve a single decision but rather require an ongoing dialogue between a practitioner, patient, and caregiver. The requirements for advance directives vary from place to place. As with financial planning, if the patient no longer has capacity to sign paperwork designating a decision maker or if there is familial discord, consultation with an eldercare attorney may be necessary to determine whether guardianship proceedings will be required. Tips for patients and their caregivers are available at the National Institute of Health's Senior Health Web site: https://nihseniorhealth.gov/endoflife/planningforcare/01.html.

Reporting Elder Abuse

> Rene calls you because Stefan appears more withdrawn and depressed since moving to the skilled nursing facility. When Rene visits, a resident tells her that one of the aides hits Stefan whenever he resists taking a bath. You call Adult Protective Services to investigate this allegation of physical abuse. After completing its investigation, Adult Protective Services determines that the physical abuse did take place and asks the institution to take corrective action. Rene decides to move her father to a different skilled nursing facility.

Acierno et al. (2010) found that 10% of 5,777 older adults reported having experienced elder abuse; this is likely an underestimate given the number of cognitively impaired and medically frail elders who are unaware or unable to report their experiences of elder abuse. Therefore, practitioners who see older adults are likely to encounter instances of elder abuse during their practice. Some common types of elder abuse are emotional abuse (causing distress through verbal or nonverbal acts), exploitation (particularly financial), and neglect (failure to provide food, shelter, clothing, health care, and basic protection). Elder abuse can occur both in the home and in institutions. If practitioners suspect abuse, they should immediately report it to local Adult Protective Services. All health care professionals are mandated reporters, and suspicion of abuse is always sufficient grounds for an investigation. The National Center on Elder Abuse, which is part of the Department of Health and Human Services, provides a wealth of information about this important topic (https://ncea.acl.gov).

CHAPTER 15

Psychotherapeutic Interventions

IN the past, mental health practitioners were taught that older patients could not participate in psychotherapy because they were too set in their ways to benefit, were unable to keep frequent appointments because of physical disability, or had cognitive impairments that prevented them from learning new skills. Research over the past few decades, however, has demonstrated that this population can indeed benefit from psychotherapy, and novel approaches, particularly for depression, have been developed specifically to accommodate the needs of older adults who may be homebound and/or have cognitive impairment (Simon et al. 2015; Wang and Blazer 2015). The importance of psychotherapy as a treatment option for older adults cannot be overstated. Because only 40%–60% of older adults experience full remission after a single antidepressant trial, practitioners should consider adjunct treatment such as psychotherapy to help their patients achieve full remission (Lenze et al. 2008; Wang and Blazer 2015). Many people do not want to take more medications or are concerned about polypharmacy; therefore, practitioners should at least be familiar with available psychotherapies so they will know how to properly refer patients. Table 15–1 lists common psychotherapies for older adults and the mental health disorders for which they are commonly used.

Supportive Therapy

Della is a 73-year-old woman with persistent depressive disorder (dysthymia) and diabetes who has failed to respond to multiple antidepressant trials. Depression interferes with

TABLE 15–1. Types of psychotherapy for older adults

Type of psychotherapy	Type of mental health disorders
Supportive psychotherapy	All types, particularly for patients with limited awareness of their mental health disorder
Psychodynamic psychotherapy	Most commonly used for depression, anxiety, and personality disorders Also used for eating, posttraumatic stress, panic, somatic symptom, and substance use disorders
Cognitive-behavioral therapy	Most commonly used for depression, anxiety, panic disorder, and insomnia Also used for psychotic, substance use, eating, and somatic symptom disorders
Interpersonal therapy (including interpersonal therapy for cognitive impairment)	Used for depression, including depression with comorbid cognitive impairment
Dialectical behavior therapy	Most commonly used for borderline personality disorder but also useful for depression with comorbid personality disorder
Problem-solving therapy	Most commonly used for depression and anxiety, including depression with comorbid cognitive impairment, and homebound older adults

Source. Francis and Kumar 2013; Wang and Blazer 2015.

her ability to follow a diabetic diet. She tells you, "I eat sugary foods whenever I feel stressed." She admits that she does not engage in physical activity regularly and states, "I just don't feel like exercising." She refuses to see a therapist because "I don't need to be brainwashed." You engage her in supportive therapy, making positive comments whenever she follows her diet and is physically active. After 1 year, Della's hemoglobin A_{1c} has improved from 10.1 to 8.6 and she is able to consistently walk 10–15 minutes each day.

Supportive therapy is probably the most commonly used type of psychotherapy because it requires neither intensive training nor a manualized approach. In supportive psychotherapy, you rarely interpret a patient's behavior but rather provide emotional support by listening sympathetically and offering encouragement for positive behaviors. Although much of the psychotherapy research literature regarding older adults emphasizes that more subspecialized psychotherapy demonstrates higher efficacy, the utility of supportive therapy should not be underestimated, especially while practitioners are building relationships with their patients (Wang and Blazer 2015).

Psychodynamic Psychotherapy

Psychodynamic psychotherapy, also known as insight-oriented psychotherapy, is a variant of classic psychoanalysis that focuses on the understanding and interpretation of unconscious processes affecting a patient's current behavior. The patient should be able to tolerate the emotional distress of discussing unresolved feelings and past conflicts that influence her behaviors in the present. Psychodynamic psychotherapy in older adults is similar to that for younger adults, although some modifications may need to be made for patients with physical impairment, mild neurocognitive disorder, or the early stages of major neurocognitive disorder (Morgan 2003). Modifications may include a mix of family sessions and confidential individual sessions rather than individual sessions alone, reviewing material from previous sessions and giving homework, and exploration of the loss of cognitive and physical abilities with age and loss of independence. One longitudinal study looking at psychodynamic psychotherapy in adults age 60 and older with mostly unipolar depressive and anxiety diagnoses demonstrated that they derived significant therapeutic benefit and did not need fewer sessions due to their age (Roseborough et al. 2013).

Cognitive-Behavioral Therapy

Cognitive-behavioral therapy (CBT) is one of the most popular psychotherapies because it is readily accessible and time limited, often 10–20 weekly sessions, and can be used in one-on-one sessions or in a group (Francis and Kumar 2013; Wang and Blazer 2015). Although therapists do need training to learn a manualized approach, practitioners should note that there are a number of "self-help" workbooks based on cognitive-behavioral techniques that can be used by patients who are independent and highly motivated (e.g., Greenberger and Padesky 2015). Unlike psychodynamic psychotherapy, CBT is focused on the present and involves learning problem-solving skills that will be useful for the rest of life. CBT is based on the belief that perception influences thoughts and, consequently, behavior. A patient learns to test whether her perception matches reality, then learns to change any misperceptions so that thoughts and eventually behavior will change (Beck Institute of Cognitive Behavior Therapy 2016).

CBT is used mostly for depressive and anxiety disorders, but studies have demonstrated its efficacy for a wide range of other disorders including, but not limited to, insomnia, substance use, schizophrenia (in conjunction with psychotropic use), eating disorders, and depression in bipolar disorder (Hofmann et al. 2012). CBT for depressive disorders in older adults has been shown to be better than treatment as usual (Gould et al. 2012), but further studies are needed to compare it with other types of psychotherapies and pharmacotherapy. CBT has also been shown to work in depression comorbid with medical and neurological disorders (Dobkin et al. 2011; Kunik et al. 2001), although some significant modifications, such as caregiver involvement and behavioral management techniques, are needed for patients with major neurocognitive disorder (Teri et al. 1997). CBT for generalized anxiety disorder in older adults is also efficacious but may require substantial changes, including homework assignments and reminder phone calls from the therapist (Mohlman et al. 2003).

Finally, the importance of CBT for insomnia (CBT-I) in older adults cannot be overemphasized. CBT-I consists of cognitive techniques to address thoughts that are preventing the patient from sleeping; guidelines for sleep hygiene, sleep restriction, and stress reduction; and relaxation exercises. Many older adults, however, also experience significant pain and other physical issues that prevent them from sleeping. Therapists should closely collaborate with practitioners to address any underlying medical issues that may disrupt sleep, such as ensuring that pain medications are taken before bedtime or switching the timing of diuretics to prevent nocturia. Even though substantial evidence exists for its efficacy, CBT-I remains highly underutilized (McCurry et al. 2007; Sivertsen et al. 2006).

Interpersonal Therapy

Interpersonal therapy (IPT) is a depression-focused psychotherapy that often appeals to older adults because its main tenets are that depression results from life events and is a medical illness, and therefore it reduces the patient's sense of being responsible for her depression (Francis and Kumar 2013; Wang and Blazer 2015). The success of IPT, however, may be decreased in adults age 70 and older, and IPT is most effective when used with pharmacotherapy (Reynolds et al. 1999a, 1999b, 2006, 2010). One small trial of IPT showed reduced depression and suicidal ideation in older adults with these conditions who were on pharmacotherapy (Heisel et al. 2015). Monthly IPT was also better than clinical care for preventing recurrence in older adults with depression and comorbid cognitive impairment (Carreira et al. 2008).

IPT for cognitive impairment (IPT-CI) focuses on role transition for patients who have depression with comorbid mild neurocognitive disorder or early major neurocognitive disorder. The therapist's goals in IPT-CI differ from those in traditional IPT in several ways (Miller and Reynolds 2007). First, instead of asking a patient to explore the positive aspects of a new role, the therapist emphasizes compensation or enhancement of the patient's remaining abilities. Second, instead of asking a patient to acquire new skills to adjust to a new role, the therapist focuses on having the patient develop relationships within her cognitive abilities and accept assistance from others when clinically indicated. Third, the therapist uses a combined patient/caregiver approach that provides psychoeducation and support to help the caregiver as the patient's needs change because of increased cognitive impairment.

Dialectical Behavior Therapy

Marsha Linehan originally designed dialectical behavior therapy (DBT) to treat borderline personality disorder (Lieb et al. 2004; Stoffers et al. 2012). The technique has been so successful that its use has spread to other mental health disorders, including depressive and eating disorders (Bankoff et al. 2012; Lynch et al. 2007). The principles of DBT are mindfulness (being aware of one's feelings; Lieb et al. 2004); distress tolerance (accepting difficult situations rather than trying to change them); interpersonal effectiveness (expressing one's feelings appropriately while respecting the feelings of others); and emotion regulation (learning to recognize and then manage one's emotions instead of being easily influenced by either positive or negative external circumstances). DBT can be helpful for geriatric patients with comorbid depression and personality disorder (Lynch 2000; Lynch et al. 2003, 2007), including those who tend to be less responsive to antidepressants. The main treatment components of DBT are a skills training group, individual therapy, phone coaching, and a therapist consultation team (Lieb et al. 2004). Despite the well-demonstrated efficacy of DBT, challenges for older patients include finding DBT-trained therapists and being willing to commit to an intensive course of treatment.

Problem-Solving Therapy

> Uri is a 66-year-old man diagnosed with major depressive disorder and mild neurocognitive disorder. A combination of maximum doses of sertraline and mirtazapine has led to only partial remission. Uri is not interested in further medication trials but is concerned about his continuing mild depressive symptoms. You discuss with him various options for depression-focused psychotherapies, including CBT, IPT, and problem-solving therapy (PST). On the basis of the availability of therapists who accept his insurance, he agrees to complete a course of PST. Uri later reports that his depressive symptoms have improved and he has made a number of positive lifestyle changes, including increasing physical activity and losing 10 pounds.

PST is another depression-focused psychotherapy that has been shown to be successful with older adults (Francis and Kumar 2013; Kiosses and Alexopoulos 2014; Wang and Blazer 2015). The premise is that people need to learn skills to solve their daily problems and decrease stress and then use these skills to deal with future problems. The efficacy of PST has been demonstrated in a wide range of populations, including home health care patients, stroke patients, patients with executive dysfunction, and patients with visual impairments (Kiosses and Alexopoulos 2014). PST has been used in primary care settings and at home via several modalities (face-to-face, telephone, Skype, and Internet) (Kiosses and Alexopoulos 2014). PST is time limited, usually lasting about 12 weeks. Variants can accommodate older adults with cognitive impairment; examples include PST for executive dysfunction and problem-adaptation therapy (PATH) for homebound elders with mild neurocognitive disorder or early major neurocognitive disorder (Alexopoulos et al. 2011; Kiosses et al. 2010).

PST is one of many different psychotherapies through which a practitioner can effectively engage and treat older adults experiencing mental distress and illness. Most of the psychotherapies employed in older adults are depression-focused psychotherapies, although CBT (and even DBT) can be modified to treat a wide range of mental health disorders. Despite the stereotype of older adults being unable to participate in psychotherapy, traditional depression-focused psychotherapies have been adapted to improve depressive symptoms and function in patients with a wide range of cognitive, physical, and functional disabilities. Many older adults with mental health disorders receive psychopharmacological instead of psychotherapeutic interventions because they have inadequate insurance coverage or cannot find trained therapists. Practitioners should actively encourage evidence-based psychotherapies whenever possible.

CHAPTER 16

Psychopharmacological Interventions

WHEN seeing younger adults, mental health practitioners often struggle to convince patients to take even a single medication as part of a treatment plan. Younger adults are not accustomed to taking medications of any kind, let alone those that can influence behavior and cognition, so clinical encounters can become variations on the theme of "take your meds." In contrast, because many older adults have become accustomed to taking multiple medications for each problem they experience, the clinical theme in work with older adults often becomes "take the right meds" or "take fewer meds."

To help guide you in striking the right balance between altering, adding, and removing the medications in an older adult's regimen, we review in this chapter some challenges of prescribing psychotropic medications in older adults, the major classes of these drugs, and considerations involved in determining when, why, and how to discontinue a medication. Our guidance is no replacement for geriatric training, years of experience, or even the knowledge presented in a complete textbook of geriatric psychopharmacology (e.g., Jacobson 2014; Salzman 2005), but we provide some of the lessons we have learned from our experience.

How Aging Affects Pharmacology

As people age, pharmacokinetic and pharmacodynamic changes typically occur in their bodies. As muscle mass decreases and peripheral fat stores increase, lipophilic drugs remain in the body longer. In addition, decreased renal clearance and hepatic blood flow combine to slow the clearance of drugs. The result is that some drug doses build up more quickly in older patients, exerting greater therapeutic and adverse effects at lower doses than expected. Alternatively, some drugs can take longer to be cleared. Therefore, if a practitioner decides to decrease a medication, assessing a patient at a lower dose can take significantly longer with an older adult than with a younger adult. Given these changes in pharmacokinetics that occur with aging, we follow the golden rule for prescribing for older adults: *start low, go slow*. Table 16–1 summarizes age-related changes affecting pharmacokinetic responses to drugs.

BASIC PRINCIPLES OF GERIATRIC PSYCHOPHARMACOLOGY

Start low. An older adult often needs only 25%–50% of the starting dose and 50%–75% of the effective dose that a younger adult requires.

Go slow. A therapeutic response to new medication often takes longer in older people.

Add one at a time. Before you prescribe a second or adjunctive medication for an older patient, titrate the first medication to the maximum tolerated dose. Avoid highly lipophilic drugs such as diazepam. Because older people have higher fat stores, highly lipophilic drugs may be erratically released.

Medication Noncompliance and Diversion

When a patient's treatment plan is not proceeding as expected, the practitioner should consider the possibility that the patient may not be taking drugs as instructed; about 20% of prescriptions are never filled, and 50% of medications are not taken as prescribed (Viswanathan et al. 2012). Practitioners should ask patients to bring in their bottles of medications to verify that they are taking the medications correctly. Older patients may not be able to follow through on a regimen for a wide range of reasons, including financial difficulties, cognitive or physical impairment, and intentional dose skipping. Even mild neurocognitive disorder can affect the patient's ability to comply with straightforward drug regimens, particularly if executive or memory dysfunction is

TABLE 16–1. Changes in pharmacokinetics secondary to aging

Process	Changes	Effects on prescribing for older adults
Gut absorption	Normal or decreased absorption if delayed gastric emptying or reduced motility	None
Permeability of blood-brain barrier	Normal or increased permeability if decreased P-glycoprotein pump function in some older adults	Possibly higher drug levels in brain
Distribution	Increased fat body stores	Longer half-life of lipophilic drugs (most psychotropics) Higher concentration for water-soluble drugs (e.g., lithium)
Metabolism	Oxidation by CYP enzymes strongly affected by aging; acetylation and methylation unchanged in normal aging	Psychotropics that are CYP substrates may be affected, depending on the type of CYP metabolizer
Clearance	Decreased renal clearance Decreased hepatic blood flow	Takes longer to achieve therapeutic blood levels Higher levels in blood once steady state achieved

Note. CYP=cytochrome P450.
Source. Adapted from Jacobson 2014.

present. Recommended approaches to address each of these problems can be found in Table 16–2.

Diversion of medications, particularly of controlled substances, is also a serious issue. Half of individuals age 12 and older who use medications for nonmedical purposes obtained psychotherapeutic drugs and pain relievers for their most recent nonmedical use from a friend or relative, and 80% or more of these users of pain relievers for nonmedical purposes stated that the patients giving away medication received all their drugs from one doctor, which defies the commonly held myth that patients have to shop with multiple practitioners to divert their medications (Substance Abuse and Mental Health Services Administration 2014). Practitioners should be aware of prescription drug misuse as a serious problem among elderly patients. It is best to minimize prescribing as-needed doses of controlled substances such as benzodiazepines, sedative-hypnotics, and stimulants to avoid the stockpiling of medications that may lead to overdoses. If practitioners suspect diversion, they should confirm whether the patients are actually taking their medications by performing an initial urine toxicology screen and confirming the results with gas chromatography/mass spectrometry. Serum drug level testing may be possible for detecting some types of medications. Random urine toxicology screens are generally more informative and minimize manipulation of results.

Failed Medication Trials

> Peter is a 77-year-old man who recently moved to be closer to his son and grandchildren. He is visiting your clinic to establish care. During routine screening, he scores 22 on the Patient Health Questionnaire 9-item depression scale (PHQ-9) and, when interviewed, acknowledges that he has been depressed for several years. He is reluctant to initiate treatment, saying, "I already tried three different antidepressants and none worked, so I just live with my depression." Peter reports that he tried citalopram for 3 days but stopped taking it because of nausea. He then tried fluoxetine for 5 days and quit taking it because "I was feeling more depressed, not less." Finally, he tried venlafaxine for 2 weeks but stopped when his anxiety worsened.

One of the challenges of prescribing psychotropic medications for older adults is that failed trials are more common

TABLE 16–2. Approaches to addressing common reasons for medication noncompliance in older adults

Problem	Potential solutions
Financial barriers/ failure to fill prescriptions	Working with pharmacists to find cheaper alternatives (e.g., 90-day supply vs. 30-day supply, splitting tablets) or cheaper medications in the same class
	Working with social services to help patient get insurance
	Working with patient to use nonpharmacological interventions such as diet and exercise to improve health status and decrease need for medications
	Participation in medication assistance programs, usually sponsored by pharmacy companies
	Pharmacy delivery programs
Cognitive impairment	Engaging others to remind patient to take medications
	Medication timers
	Timed pillboxes, pillbox organizers
	Written directions
	Coordinating pill taking with meals/ bedtime/daily routines
Physical impairment	Non-childproof containers
	Blister packs
	Talking medication containers
	Large-print labels
	Easy-to-break tablets
Intentional dose skipping	Education directed toward patient decision making
	Practitioner use of open, collaborative communication style in discussing medications with patients

Source. Adapted from Marek and Antle 2008.

among older patients, who have more adverse reactions and higher rates of treatment-resistant depression than the general adult population. We briefly discuss the management of failed medication trials for each category of drugs in the following section, "Classes of Psychotropic Medications Commonly Used With Older Adults." In general, practitioners should attempt adequate trials of at least two or three lower-price generic psychotropic medications, preferably ones that have different drug mechanisms, before trying a more expensive generic or brand-name psychotropic. Practitioners should also make sure to carefully document the trial of each psychotropic to provide helpful information when referring more complex patients to mental health practitioners. Documentation should include the maximum dose achieved, the length of time the patient was treated at the maximum dose, and the reason for stopping the treatment (e.g., lack of efficacy, undesirable side effect, life-threatening side effect).

Several factors can result in failed medication trials. A patient's report of a failed medication trial may actually be a report of noncompliance. A failed trial can also be due to the expense of medications. In an effort to save money, many older adults leave prescriptions unfilled, skip doses, or terminate medications prematurely. Adverse effects, both real and perceived, can also result in medication failure. Psychological factors such as the stigma of mental health treatment, preoccupation with adverse effects, or somatic preoccupation can lead a patient to perceive adverse effects that can be resolved only when a practitioner provides education and reassurance. Practitioners often neglect the importance of psychological factors—what is often called the *placebo effect*—when prescribing a medication. Practitioners need to remember that the prescription of a medication has both implicit and explicit effects on a patient, so they should consider its potential psychological effects. In addition, a patient may erroneously attribute symptoms of mental or physical illness to a psychotropic. For example, a patient may attribute a tremor to a medication when he is actually showing the first signs of Parkinson's disease, or a patient may report that the first dose of a selective serotonin reuptake inhibitor (SSRI) deepened his depression because he had unrealistic expectations about how the medication works. Prescribing a medication to a patient is only the first step in actually delivering its benefits.

Classes of Psychotropic Medications Commonly Used With Older Adults

DEPRESSIVE DISORDER TREATMENTS

Peter has already failed several medication trials for depression, so he has an increased risk of failing another trial. Concerned, you ask Peter about successful medication trials. He tells you that he once took diazepam and describes it as a "magic pill." He wants any new medication you prescribe to work just as quickly. You discuss the known efficacy and adverse effects of treatments for depression, including initial gastrointestinal effects and the delay between initiating treatment and symptom response. Peter acknowledges anxiety about taking any psychotropic medication because "it will make me look weak." His budget is also tight, and he is worried about the cost. He agrees to try sertraline because it is the cheapest medication on his prescription formulary. You promise to "start low and go slow" so that Peter can immediately report any side effects that he is experiencing. He eventually agrees to try sertraline at 12.5 mg/day, which he tolerates well, and then agrees to a very slow dose increase to 50 mg/day over the course of 6 weeks. After Peter has taken sertraline 50 mg/day for 2 months, his PHQ-9 score decreases to 13, and he reports subjective improvement of his mental health symptoms. Peter says he does not want to take a higher dose of sertraline because he fears becoming addicted. Despite your multiple attempts to explain that depressive disorder treatments, unlike benzodiazepines, are not habit forming, Peter refuses to consider a higher dose. Therefore, you recommend cognitive-behavioral therapy (CBT) to help achieve full remission of his depressive symptoms. After Peter completes the course of CBT, his PHQ-9 score drops to 3, and he denies any depression during his clinical interview. Following 9 months of persistent work, Peter's depressive symptoms are now in full remission.

The medications that are commonly used to treat depressive disorders are listed in Table 16–3. The classes of first-line treatments for depression include SSRIs, serotonin-norepinephrine reuptake inhibitors (SNRIs), norepinephrine and dopamine reuptake inhibitors, and α_2-adrenergic and serotonergic antagonists. Tricyclic antidepressants (TCAs) and monoamine oxidase inhibitors (MAOIs) are second-line treatments because of their adverse-effect profiles (including anticholinergic side effects for TCAs and dietary restrictions for MAOIs) and the

TABLE 16–3. Depressive disorder treatments commonly used in older adults

Drug	Recommended starting and target doses	Special concerns
SSRIs		
Citalopram	Starting; 10 mg/day Target: 10–20 mg/day	FDA black box warning recommends not to exceed 20 mg/day in people older than age 60 or who have a history of stroke or cardiac disease
Escitalopram	Starting; 5–10 mg/day Target: 5–20 mg/day	Enantiomer of citalopram FDA black box warning recommends not to exceed 20 mg/day in people older than age 60 or who have a history of stroke or cardiac disease
Fluoxetine	Starting; 5–10 mg/day Target: 5–40 mg/day (60 mg/day for OCD)	Long half-life compared with other SSRIs; needs washout period of 5 weeks before starting TCAs or MAOIs
Paroxetine	Starting; 5–10 mg/day Target: 5–40 mg/day (60 mg/day for OCD) CR starting: 12.5 mg/day CR target: 12.5–50 mg/day	Short-half life Possible anticholinergic side effects
Sertraline	Starting: 12.5–25 mg/day Target: 25–200 mg/day (higher in OCD)	

TABLE 16–3. Depressive disorder treatments commonly used in older adults *(continued)*

Drug	Recommended starting and target doses	Special concerns
SNRIs		
Desvenlafaxine	Starting: 50 mg qod Target: 50 mg qod or 50 mg/day	Active metabolite of venlafaxine Discontinue medication gradually to prevent withdrawal symptoms
Duloxetine	Starting: 20 mg/day Target: 20–60 mg/day	Minimize use in patients with end-stage renal disease or hepatic insufficiency FDA approval for neuropathic pain and fibromyalgia Discontinue medication gradually to prevent withdrawal symptoms Lab monitoring: liver function tests at baseline and then as clinically indicated
Levomilnacipran	XR starting: 20 mg/day XR target: 40–120 mg/day	FDA approval in 2013 for MDD Limited data in older adults Discontinue medication gradually to prevent withdrawal symptoms

TABLE 16–3. Depressive disorder treatments commonly used in older adults *(continued)*

Drug	Recommended starting and target doses	Special concerns
Milnacipran	Starting: 12.5 mg/day Target: 50–200 mg/day	FDA approval for fibromyalgia, but its enantiomer (levomilnacipran) has FDA approval for depression Discontinue medication gradually to prevent withdrawal symptoms
Venlafaxine	IR starting: 25 mg bid IR target: 150–225 mg/day (bid or tid dosing) XR starting; 37.5 mg/day XR target: 150–225 mg/day (once-daily dosing)	XR form preferable to IR to prevent withdrawal symptoms Missing doses (particularly IR) can cause unpleasant withdrawal symptoms Discontinue medication gradually to prevent withdrawal symptoms
TCAs		
Desipramine	Starting: 25 mg/day Target: 25–150 mg/day	Therapeutic serum level >115 ng/mL; potential toxicity at >300 ng/mL
Nortriptyline	Starting: 10 mg/day Target: 10–100 mg/day	Therapeutic serum level 50–150 ng/mL

TABLE 16–3. Depressive disorder treatments commonly used in older adults *(continued)*

Drug	Recommended starting and target doses	Special concerns
MAOIs		
Selegiline (transdermal)	Starting: 6 mg/day Target: 6–12 mg/day	No dietary restrictions at 6 mg/day (or 2 weeks after reducing dosage from 12 to 6 mg/day) Hold patch at least 10 days prior to elective surgery with general anesthesia
Other classes		
Bupropion (IR, SR, XL formulations)	IR starting: 37.5–75 mg qam IR target: 75–225 mg/day SR starting: 100 mg qam SR target: 100–300 mg/day XL starting: 150 mg qam XL target: 150–300 mg/day	Norepinephrine and dopamine reuptake inhibitor Low risk of seizure (<0.5%) for dosages ≤450 mg/day
Mirtazapine	Starting: 7.5 mg qhs Target: 7.5–45 mg/day	α_2-Adrenergic inhibitor Histaminergic properties at low doses (sedation, increased appetite)
St. John's wort	Starting 300 mg tid Target: 300 mg tid	Do not take concurrently with serotonergic medications (e.g., SSRIs, SNRIs, MAOIs)

TABLE 16–3. Depressive disorder treatments commonly used in older adults *(continued)*

Drug	Recommended starting and target doses	Special concerns
Trazodone	Insomnia Starting: 25 mg qhs Target: 25–50 mg qhs Depression Starting: 75 mg qhs Target: 75–375 mg qhs	$5\text{-HT}_{2A/2C}$ and α_1-adrenergic antagonist Mainly used as off-label treatment for insomnia because target doses used for depression cause sedation
Vilazodone	Starting: 10 mg/day Target: 20–40 mg/day	Selective 5-HT reuptake inhibitor and 5-HT_{1A} partial agonist FDA approval in 2011 for MDD Limited data in older adults
Vortioxetine	Starting: 10 mg/day Target: 20–40 mg/day	Multiple effects on 5-HT receptors (partial 5-HT_{1B} receptor agonism, 5-HT_7 antagonism, 5-HT_3 antagonism); inhibition of the 5-HT transporter

Note. 5-HT=serotonin; bid=twice daily; CR=controlled release; FDA=U.S. Food and Drug Administration; IR=immediate release; MAOI=monoamine oxidase inhibitor; MDD=major depressive disorder; OCD=obsessive-compulsive disorder; qam=every morning; qhs=every night; qod=every other day; SNRI=serotonin-norepinephrine reuptake inhibitor; SR=sustained release; SSRI=selective serotonin reuptake inhibitor; TCA=tricyclic antidepressant; tid=three times daily; XL=extended release; XR=extended release.
Source. Asnis and Henderson 2015; Croft et al. 2014; Davidson 1989; Gury and Cousin 1999; Jacobson 2014; Laughren et al. 2011; U.S. Food and Drug Administration 2011.

higher likelihood of lethality if patients overdose on them. In general, the first-line treatments have similar efficacy (e.g., Fournier et al. 2010). The decision to use a first-line treatment is based on several factors, including tolerability by the patient; the potential for dual benefits (e.g., duloxetine to treat both major depressive disorder and diabetic neuropathy), which helps minimize polypharmacy; better adverse-effect profile; and cost.

The rule to *start low, go slow* is especially important when treating depression. Many older adults will discontinue SSRIs or SNRIs because of adverse gastrointestinal effects, even though the effects can be minimized by taking the medication with food and typically resolve during the first week or two of treatment. Some older adults experience paradoxical anxiety if an SSRI or SNRI is started at too high a dose or titrated too quickly.

Because only about 50% of older adults respond adequately to an optimal trial of a first-line treatment (Lenze et al. 2008), practitioners often need to consider a course of psychotherapy, the initiation of electroconvulsive therapy, or the addition of a second or adjunctive psychotropic medication. The National Institute of Mental Health–funded Sequenced Treatment Alternatives to Relieve Depression (STAR*D) trial, which included patients from both mental health and primary care settings, studied how those who failed to respond to a previous treatment for depression responded to a subsequent treatment. Although the STAR*D study examined the general adult population, many of its findings are useful for older adults. Some of the major findings were that 1) full response can take as long as 10–12 weeks; 2) with every additional treatment required to treat depression, the likelihood of success decreased; 3) patients who had full remission did better than those who had partial remission of their depressive symptoms; and 4) patients who needed more than one treatment attempt were more likely to have severe depressive symptoms and comorbid psychiatric and medical problems (National Institute of Mental Health 2006). Given these results, practitioners in primary care should discuss with their patients how long it can take to respond to depressive disorder treatments and caution that more than one trial may be needed to treat depression effectively.

BIPOLAR DISORDER TREATMENTS

Treatments studied for bipolar disorder can be used in older adults to treat various mental health symptoms, including but not limited to manic symptoms due to primary psychiatry disorder and secondary causes, depressive symptoms in bipolar disorder, and mood dysregulation. Most agents, except lithium, were first studied and approved for the treatment of seizure disorders. Because these medications have multiple potential indications, it is important for a practitioner to document the specific indication for each medication—for example, epilepsy, neuropathic pain, or mood instability—so that other practitioners will know why each medication has been prescribed before electing to continue or discontinue it. In general, these medications should be carefully titrated up and down, because abrupt discontinuation can result in withdrawal seizures.

As a general rule, lithium and valproic acid are first-line treatments for bipolar disorders. Among older adults with bipolar disorder, lithium is efficacious but is difficult to take because of its narrow therapeutic index, the number of drug-drug interactions (especially with thiazide diuretics and nonsteroidal anti-inflammatory drugs), and its adverse effects (renal impairment, tremor, and cognitive dysfunction). Because of these difficulties, many geriatric mental health practitioners prefer to use valproic acid when treating patients with bipolar disorders. If valproic acid is not efficacious or cannot be tolerated, second-line treatments include levetiracetam, lamotrigine, and carbamazepine, all of which present a number of challenges. They require careful titration upward, and therefore, therapeutic effects can take longer. In particular, lamotrigine also has a number of drug-drug interactions, which affect its titration schedule. The titration schedule must be carefully followed because of the known risk of Stevens-Johnson syndrome (Table 16–4). Carbamazepine causes autoinduction of cytochrome P450 (CYP) 3A4, inducing CYP3A4 but also a substrate of CYP3A4, which can result in reduced efficacy 2–3 weeks after a stable dose is achieved.

Although a non–mental health practitioner may feel comfortable beginning an initial treatment for bipolar disorder, the treatment of an older adult with a manic, hypomanic, or bipolar depression is often complicated. For example, practitioners should be aware of the drugs that may interact with lamotrigine (Table 16–5) and should carefully review the la-

TABLE 16–4. Bipolar disorder treatments commonly used in older adults

Drug	Recommended starting and target doses	Therapeutic serum level	Special concerns
Carbamazepine	Starting: 100 mg bid Target: 200–800 mg/day (divided bid)	4–12 µg/mL	Because of anticholinergic effects, should be reserved as a last-line treatment Autoinduction may lower levels after 2–3 weeks of treatment, so dose may need to be increased Slow titration upward to decrease likelihood of Stevens-Johnson syndrome Start at 100–200 mg/day and then increase at weekly intervals on the basis of observed symptoms Can also be used for seizure management Lab monitoring: serum level at baseline and then 2–4 weeks later to monitor for autoinduction; CBC, basic metabolic panel including blood urea nitrogen and creatinine, LFTs at baseline and then every 3–12 months as clinically indicated

TABLE 16–4. Bipolar disorder treatments commonly used in older adults *(continued)*

Drug	Recommended starting and target doses	Therapeutic serum level	Special concerns
Divalproex (valproate, valproic acid)	Starting: 125–250 mg qd to bid Target: 250–1,500 mg/day (divided bid, except XR is dosed once daily)	65–90 µg/mL	Adjustment phase: VPA levels every 1–2 weeks CBCs, LFTs every 4 weeks for first 2 months Maintenance phase: depakote every 3 months; CBCs, LFTs every 6 months Can also be used for seizure management
Lamotrigine	Starting: 25 mg qd or qod (see special concerns) Target: 100–200 mg/day	Therapeutic serum level for psychiatric disorder unknown	Increase by 25–50 mg/day every 2 weeks Slow titration upward to decrease likelihood of Stevens-Johnson syndrome (see Table 16–5) Stevens-Johnson syndrome usually occurs within 2–8 week of initiation; lamotrigine should be stopped at the first sign of any rash, even if it appears benign Therapeutic dosage sensitive to drug-drug interactions (see Table 16–5) Can also be used for seizure management
Levetiracetam	Starting: 250 mg bid Target: 250–1,500 mg/day (divided bid or tid)	Therapeutic serum level for psychiatric disorder unknown	Some evidence for anti-manic behavior in dementia Increase by 250–500 mg/day every week Can also be used for seizure management

TABLE 16–4. Bipolar disorder treatments commonly used in older adults *(continued)*

Drug	Recommended starting and target doses	Therapeutic serum level	Special concerns
Lithium	Starting: 75–150 mg qhs Target: 150–1,800 mg/day (usually 300–900 mg/day)	0.4–1.0 mEq/L	Therapeutic benefit and toxicity may occur at lower serum levels in older adults because of changes in blood-brain barrier
			Educate patients about interactions with drugs, especially common over-the-counter drugs, and importance of maintaining consistent salt intake and hydration
			Consider more frequent lab monitoring in patients with large fluid shifts or renal insufficiency (lithium is renally cleared)
			Consider MedicAlert bracelet for patients who take lithium
			Lab monitoring: first lithium level after steady state achieved (usually 5 days), then every 3–12 months as clinically indicated; ECG, blood urea nitrogen, creatinine, and thyroid-stimulating hormone at baseline and then every 3–12 months as clinically indicated

Note. bid=twice daily; CBC=complete blood count; ECG=electrocardiogram; LFT=liver function test; qd=every day; qhs=at bedtime; qod=every other day; tid=three times daily; VPA=valproate; XR=extended release.
Source. Cullison et al. 2014; GlaxoSmithKline 2015; Jacobson 2014. Novartis 2015.

TABLE 16–5. Adjustments for starting dose and titration schedule for patients taking drugs that interact with lamotrigine

	Patients not taking carbamazepine, phenytoin, phenobarbital, primidone, or valproic acid	Patients taking valproic acid	Patients taking carbamazepine, phenytoin, phenobarbital, or primidone but not valproic acid
Effect on lamotrigine	None	Increases lamotrigine levels	Decreases lamotrigine levels
Adjustments for starting dose and titration schedule of lamotrigine	Follow standard titration schedule for lamotrigine Starting dose: 25 mg/day Ending dose: 200 mg/day at week 7	Decrease starting dose of lamotrigine by 50% (25 mg every other day) and slow the titration schedule by 50% (100 mg/day at week 7)	Increase starting dose of lamotrigine by 50% (50 mg/day) and speed up the titration schedule by 50% (400 mg/day at week 7)

Source. Adapted from GlaxoSmithKline 2015.

motrigine drug insert for how certain drugs may affect the lamotrigine initiation and titration schedule (GlaxoSmithKline 2015). In addition, many patients who have bipolar disorder as a primary psychiatric disorder are often noncompliant with treatment, so more intensive mental health services may be needed to ensure that they remain stable.

PSYCHOTIC DISORDER TREATMENTS

Treatments for schizophrenia and other psychotic disorders are often called "antipsychotics," but leading psychiatrists prefer to describe them on the basis of their mechanism of action (Zohar et al. 2014). Naming these medications by their mechanism of action helps practitioners understand why they are efficacious both for the treatment of psychotic disorders and as adjunctive medications for depressive, anxiety, and bipolar disorders. In Table 16–6, we review the commonly prescribed medications to treat psychotic disorders, including special concerns for their administration to older adults. Most treatments for psychotic disorders antagonize the dopamine type 2 (D_2) receptor, but many newer medications antagonize the D_2 receptor and modulate the serotonin (5-HT) receptors by acting as partial agonists at the 5-HT_{1A} receptor and antagonists at the 5-HT_{2A} receptor. These additional actions may ameliorate some of the undesirable side effects seen with medications that primarily antagonize the D_2 receptor, such as tardive dyskinesia and extrapyramidal symptoms (Meltzer 2013).

When practitioners prescribe a medication that antagonizes the D_2 receptor, they should understand which mental health symptoms or disorders they are targeting and how long they anticipate prescribing the medication. This is important not only for communication among all practitioners involved in a patient's care but also to determine whether a psychotic disorder treatment can be tapered or discontinued. It is crucial to be vigilant about psychotic disorder treatments, which may have significant adverse effects in all adults but especially in older adults.

Most practitioners are aware that medications that antagonize the D_2 receptors are associated with a higher risk of tardive dyskinesia and extrapyramidal symptoms. Medications that antagonize the D_2 receptor and modulate the 5-HT receptors are associated with metabolic syndrome and require special monitoring. Measurements that should be obtained at baseline,

TABLE 16–6. Psychotic disorder treatments commonly used in older adults

Drug	Recommended starting and target doses	Special concerns
Aripiprazole	Tablet or solution starting: 2–5 mg/day Tablet or solution target: 2–20 mg/day LAI starting: 400 mg IM every 4 weeks LAI target: 300–400 mg IM every 4 weeks	LAI not well studied in elderly and should not be used in those with dementia Initial dose for LAI should be 400 mg, but dose can be decreased to 300 mg if adverse reaction occurs
Asenapine	Starting: 5 mg bid Target: 5 mg/day to 10 mg bid	Newer medication with only one small study of asenapine in older adults with bipolar disorder (Scheidemantel et al. 2015)
Clozapine	Starting: 6.25–12.5 mg/day Target: 7.25–400 mg/day Increase 25–50 mg/day for first 2 weeks, and then no more than 100 mg 1–2 times per week	Weekly CBCs to monitor for leukopenia unless ANC <1,500/µL (see Clozapine REMS Web site for more details [https://www.clozapinerems.com]) Usually reserved for patients with psychotic disorders refractory to other treatments Side effects include agranulocytosis, seizures, myocarditis, orthostatic hypotension
Fluphenazine	Oral starting: 1–2.5 mg/day Target: 0.25–4 mg/day (divided)	Depot form available

DSM-5® Pocket Guide for Elder Mental Health

TABLE 16–6. Psychotic disorder treatments commonly used in older adults *(continued)*

Drug	Recommended starting and target doses	Special concerns
Haloperidol	Oral starting: 0.25–0.5 mg qd to tid; target: 0.25–4 mg qd IV formulation reserved for settings with telemetry Decanoate starting: 25 mg/month Decanoate target: 25–100 mg/month	Depot form available
Iloperidone	Starting: 1 mg bid Target: 6–12 mg bid	Titration packet available Not well studied in elderly Orthostatic hypotension
Lurasidone	Starting: 40 mg/day Target: 40–80 mg/day	Two studies in older adults (Forester et al. 2015; Sajatovic et al. 2016)
Olanzapine	Oral starting: 2.5 mg/day Oral target: 2.5–15 mg/day LAI starting: 150 mg im every 4 weeks LAI target: 150–300 mg im every 4 weeks	LAI not well studied in elderly and should be avoided because of risk of postinjection delirium (a side effect unique to olanzapine LAI) (Rauch and Fleischhacker 2013)

TABLE 16–6. Psychotic disorder treatments commonly used in older adults *(continued)*

Drug	Recommended starting and target doses	Special concerns
Paliperidone	XR starting: 3 mg/day XR target: 3–12 mg/day LAI starting; 156 mg IM every 4 weeks LAI target: 39–234 mg every 4 weeks	Therapeutic serum level: 3.5–50 ng/mL One small study in older adults (Tzimos et al. 2008)
Perphenazine	Starting: 2–4 mg qd to bid Target: 2–32 mg/day	Poor CYP D26 metabolizers Patients taking CYP D26 inhibitors (e.g., TCAs, SSRIs) may have higher plasma levels (Schering Corporation 2002)
Quetiapine	IR tablets starting: 12.5–50 mg qhs IR tablets target: 12.5–400 mg (divided bid to tid) XR tablets starting: 50 mg qhs XR tablets target: 50–400 mg qhs	Orthostatic hypotension Plasma levels may increase when quetiapine is administered with CYP 3A inhibitors (e.g., ketoconazole, erythromycin) (AstraZeneca 2003)
Risperidone	Oral starting: 0.25–0.5 mg qhs Oral target: 0.25–3 mg qd or bid LAI starting: 25 mg IM every 2 weeks LAI target: 12.5–50 mg IM every 2 weeks	Limited studies support efficacy of LAI in older adults with schizophrenia (Catalán and Penadés 2011)

TABLE 16–6. Psychotic disorder treatments commonly used in older adults *(continued)*

Drug	Recommended starting and target doses	Special concerns
Ziprasidone	Oral starting: 20 mg bid Oral target: 20–80 mg bid	Rare but serious skin reaction known as drug reaction with eosinophilia and systemic symptoms (DRESS) (U.S. Food and Drug Administration 2014a)

Note. ANC=absolute neutrophil count; bid=twice daily; CBC=complete blood count; CYP=cytochrome P450; im=intramuscular; IR=immediate release; IV=intravenous; LAI=long-acting injectable; qd=every day; qhs=every night; REMS=Risk Evaluation and Mitigation Strategy; tid=three times daily; XR=extended release; SSRIs=selective serotonin reuptake inhibitors; TCAs=tricyclic antidepressants.

Consider QTc monitoring for patients on both typical and atypical antipsychotics if they have a number of risk factors for QTc prolongation (e.g., history of cardiac arrhythmias).

Source. Clozapine REMS Program 2014; Jacobson 2014.

12 weeks, and annually are body mass index (BMI), waist circumference, blood pressure, fasting glucose/hemoglobin A_{1c}, and lipids. BMI should also be measured at 4 weeks, 8 weeks, and then every 3 months (American Diabetes Association et al. 2004).

Fewer practitioners are aware that all medications that antagonize the D_2 receptors increase risk of stroke, QTc prolongation that predisposes to the potentially life-threatening torsades de pointes, and sudden death (Ray et al. 2009) or that these medications are associated with cognitive decline when prescribed to patients with dementia (Vigen et al. 2011). Practitioners should discuss and document these serious adverse effects with patients. Given the overall concerns regarding adverse effects and alterations in metabolism in older adults, long-acting injectable versions should be reserved mainly for patients with chronic psychotic disorders living in the community who have demonstrated noncompliance; they should not be used in patients who have dementia with behavioral disturbances.

Finally, clozapine deserves special attention. Clozapine is an underutilized treatment for persons with psychotic disorders (Stroup et al. 2016), but prescribing it is complicated because of the risk of serious adverse effects, especially agranulocytosis, and the associated requirement for gradual titration and discontinuation. In the United States, all practitioners who prescribe clozapine and all pharmacists who dispense it are required to register in the Clozapine REMS Program. The monitoring guidelines for patients before they start and while they are taking clozapine, as well as the indications for discontinuation versus more intensive monitoring when neutropenia develops, have now been standardized by the Clozapine REMS Program. Information is available on the Clozapine REMS Web site (https://www.clozapinerems.com).

ANXIETY AND SLEEP-WAKE DISORDER TREATMENTS

Older adults frequently present for treatment of anxiety and insomnia. In the past, practitioners typically prescribed benzodiazepines to older adults experiencing anxiety and insomnia, but accumulating evidence suggests that these drugs are associated with a higher risk of falls and dementia (Woolcott et al. 2009). Today, practitioners should work to minimize the use of benzodiazepines in older adults and to discontinue their use among older adults who have become both physiologically and psychologically dependent on these medications. We discuss recommendations for tapering benzodiazepines in the next section, "Medication Discontinuation in Older Adults."

Buspirone and the psychotherapies described in Chapter 15, "Psychotherapeutic Interventions," are safer alternatives to benzodiazepines in older adults. Benzodiazepine derivatives are also commonly used as hypnotics in older adults. Z-drugs (e.g., zolpidem, zaleplon, zopiclone) are similar to benzodiazepines and have the same long-term concerns about dependence. Medications that act on other receptors, such as ramelteon, a melatonin receptor agonist, and suvorexant, an orexin receptor antagonist, need further studies in older adults. Ramelteon appears to have the potential to prevent delirium (Hatta et al. 2014). Doxepin at low doses (3–6 mg) is also approved for insomnia and can be useful for older adults (Rojas-Fernandez and Chen 2014). Practitioners should work up patients for sleep-wake disorders, particularly obstructive sleep apnea; review sleep hygiene guidelines; and refer patients for CBT for insomnia (CBT-I). In Table 16–7, we review commonly used treatments and discuss special concerns for their use among older adults.

Medication Discontinuation in Older Adults: Stopping the Epidemic of Polypharmacy

After being stable on sertraline for a year, Peter brings up the topic of discontinuing it. You express concern because he has persistent depressive disorder and probably has had at least one other major depressive episode. He insists, however, so you agree to lower his sertraline dose to 37.5 mg/ day for 3 months to see how he does. Two months later Peter reports slightly worsening depressive symptoms, and his PHQ-9 score increases to 10. He requests to participate in CBT booster sessions, which help slightly. After extensive discussion, Peter agrees to continue taking sertraline 37.5 mg/day, although he indicates he would still rather stop it completely. Although he acknowledges that his depressive symptoms were better controlled when he was taking sertraline 50 mg/ day, he insists that he would rather take a lower dose "because I feel less dependent on my medication to get through life." He takes up yoga and daily walking as adjunctive treatments for depression.

TABLE 16–7. Anxiety and sleep-wake disorder treatments commonly used in older adults[a]

Drug	Recommended starting and target doses	Special concerns
Buspirone	Starting: 5 mg bid Target: 5 mg bid to 20 mg tid	
Doxepin (low-dose)[a]	Starting: 3 mg qhs Target: 3–6 mg qhs	Less likely to have anticholinergic effects at low doses
Eszopiclone	Starting: Difficulty with sleep initiation 1 mg; difficulty with sleep maintenance 2 mg Target:1–2 mg qhs	
Gabapentin	Starting: Anxiety: 100 mg every 12 hours; insomnia 100 mg qhs Target: Anxiolytic effect 200–1,800 mg/day; insomnia 100–300 mg qhs	Has FDA approval only for neuralgia and epilepsy; use for anxiety or insomnia is off-label
Lorazepam[a]	Starting: Anxiety 0.25–0.5 mg qd to bid; insomnia 0.25–0.5 mg qhs Target: 0.25–2 mg/day	
Melatonin	Starting: 0.5–6 mg/qhs (within 30–120 minutes of bedtime) Target: 1–6 mg/qhs	FDA considers melatonin to be a dietary supplement, not a drug

TABLE 16–7. Anxiety and sleep-wake disorder treatments commonly used in older adults[a] *(continued)*

Drug	Recommended starting and target doses	Special concerns
Ramelteon	Starting: 8 mg (within 30 minutes of bedtime) Target: 8 mg (within 30 minutes of bedtime) Mechanism: melatonin receptor agonist	Limited evidence for preventive use in delirium (Hatta et al. 2014)
Suvorexant	Starting: 10 mg qhs Target: 10–40 mg qhs Mechanism: orexin receptor antagonist	Limited knowledge about effects in elderly Unlike benzodiazepines and Z-drugs, suvorexant has no known effects in mild to moderate obstructive sleep apnea (Sun et al. 2016)
Zaleplon[a]	Starting: 5 mg qhs Target: 5–10 mg immediately before bedtime	

TABLE 16–7. Anxiety and sleep-wake disorder treatments commonly used in older adults[a] (continued)

Drug	Recommended starting and target doses	Special concerns
Zolpidem[a]	Starting: IR 5 mg qhs CR: 6.25 mg immediately before bedtime Target: IR 5–10 mg qhs CR: 6.25–12.5 mg qhs	Lower doses for women because they are at higher risk for neuropsychiatric effects (hallucinations/sensory distortion, amnesia, sleepwalking, and nocturnal eating) Zolpidem is the psychotropic drug most commonly implicated in emergency department visits for adverse medication events in older adults (Hampton et al. 2014) Assess for motor impairment, particularly in patients who are driving FDA advises against next-day driving in patients taking Ambien CR (U.S. Food and Drug Administration 2016)

Note. bid=twice daily; CR=controlled release; FDA=U.S. Food and Drug Administration; IR=immediate release; qd=every day; qhs=every night; tid=three times daily.
[a]Benzodiazepines and Z-drugs should be used with caution because of the risks of increased falls and dementia. These should ideally be prescribed on a short-term basis except in rare circumstances such as end-of-life or palliative care cases.
Source. Bennett et al. 2014; Jacobson 2014; U.S. Food and Drug Administration 2014b, 2016.

Polypharmacy leads to two-thirds of older adult emergency department visits (Budnitz et al. 2011). It increases the likelihood of nursing home placement, poorer functioning, high mortality rates, and higher hospitalizations rates (Garfinkel and Mangin 2010). Knowing when and how to discontinue medications is just as important a skill as prescribing them.

When deciding whether to discontinue a patient's psychotropic medication, the practitioner should consider the following four discontinuation indications:

1. *The risk of a psychotropic outweighs its benefits.* This is the case, for example, when a patient prescribed zolpidem falls during a sleepwalking episode and sustains a subarachnoid hemorrhage.
2. *A psychotropic may be replaced by a safer alternative.* Examples are when a benzodiazepine can be replaced with melatonin for sleep or an antihistaminergic can be replaced with sleep hygiene techniques.
3. *Although a psychotropic provides some benefit on its own, its risks are unacceptable in the setting of polypharmacy and the resulting adverse effects from drug-drug interactions.* This situation is often due to communication breakdown, which occurs when multiple practitioners prescribe medications for the same patient without coordinating care or being aware of potential drug-drug interactions. An example is when a psychiatrist prescribes an SSRI for depression, a neurologist prescribes a TCA for neuropathic pain, and a primary care practitioner then adds tramadol for lower back pain. Although each of these medications may be effective, the patient is at increased risk for adverse effects such as serotonin syndrome.
4. *An adjunctive psychotropic is no longer needed.* For example, a patient with bipolar disorder requires the prescription of a D_2 antagonist in addition to his usual valproic acid. After his mania remits, it is reasonable to gradually discontinue the D_2 antagonist.

Each of these discontinuation indications requires different strategic approaches:

1. When the risks of a medication outweigh its benefits, the practitioner should discontinue the medication as quickly as possible. The major exception is benzodiaze-

pines; successful tapers of benzodiazepines in patients who have been relying on those medications can be challenging and may require the involvement of a mental health practitioner.

2. When a medication may be replaced with a safer alternative, a practitioner should broach the subject of discontinuing it in the context of offering a replacement. It is always important to offer an alternative form of assistance, but doing so is especially critical if a patient may have developed a physical or psychological dependence on a medication such as a benzodiazepine.

3. When polypharmacy is occurring, all the practitioners prescribing medications to a patient should engage in a dialogue about his various medications. They need to build consensus on reducing polypharmacy. Patient and caregiver must also play a proactive role in medication management to understand the purpose of the medications, raise concerns about adverse effects with their practitioners, and insist that practitioners communicate with each other. In this situation, there needs to be a "quarterback," usually the primary care practitioner or geriatric medicine consultant, who will be the final decision maker, particularly when two subspecialists have conflicting opinions about whether a medication should be continued.

4. When an adjunctive psychotropic is no longer needed, it usually helps to seek consultation from a mental health practitioner. This is especially true if a patient is taking multiple psychotropics or has a severe mental illness, such as a bipolar or psychotic disorder. Collaborative discussions between primary care and mental health practitioners, ideally within an integrated setting, are most likely to produce the best balance of medical and mental health benefits. In this scenario, clinical assessment after each dose reduction can be helpful in determining how quickly the taper can occur.

Table 16–8 describes considerations and alternatives for medications for various disorders.

TABLE 16–8. Medication discontinuation

Medication	Diagnosis or disorder	First-line or safer alternatives	Special considerations for medication discontinuation
Medications for depressive disorders	Major depressive disorder, single episode	Consider CBT if patient is cognitively intact or other types of depression-focused psychotherapies	Consult with mental health practitioner prior to discontinuation of medications if patient has other comorbid psychiatric disorders, previously had severe mental health symptoms (e.g., suicidality or psychosis), or required inpatient psychiatric hospitalization or electroconvulsive therapy. Consider mental health consultation for patient who has had previous depressive episodes.
Medications for bipolar disorders	Manic episodes	Consider CBT, IPSRT, family-focused psychotherapy, and psychoeducation; these treatments should be used in conjunction with medications	Consider mental health consultation before medication discontinuation. Slowly taper bipolar disorder treatment over months to years.
Medications for psychotic disorders	Delirium	Nonpharmacological approaches for delirium (e.g., reorientation)	Inform caregiver of the need to discontinue D_2 antagonist posthospitalization. Discontinue D_2 antagonist within days to weeks once delirium resolves.

TABLE 16–8. Medication discontinuation (continued)

Medication	Diagnosis or disorder	First-line or safer alternatives	Special considerations for medication discontinuation
Medications for psychotic disorders (continued)	Dementia with agitation	Nonpharmacological approaches for first-line treatment for agitation Consider off-label use of SSRIs, SNRIs, or valproic acid for agitation, particularly in dementia	Consider discontinuation for mild cases to see if nonpharmacological management alone works. More severe cases of agitation may benefit from mental health consultation before discontinuation.
	Dementia with psychotic symptoms (e.g., paranoia, delusions)	Nonpharmacological approaches for first-line treatment for psychosis (redirection, empathetic but noncommittal responses)	Consider discontinuation for mild cases to see if nonpharmacological management alone works. More severe cases of psychosis may benefit from mental health consultation before discontinuation.
	Schizophrenia lasting at least several months	Consider CBT for psychosis if patient is cognitively intact, but CBT needs to be used with medications to treat schizophrenia	Consult with mental health practitioner before attempting dose reduction. Highly stable patients should be considered for reduction if dosing is higher than geriatric doses.

TABLE 16–8. Medication discontinuation (*continued*)

Medication	Diagnosis or disorder	First-line or safer alternatives	Special considerations for medication discontinuation
Medications for anxiety and sleep-wake disorders	Depressive and anxiety disorders	Consider CBT and/or antidepressants (e.g., SSRIs or SNRIs)	Provide psychoeducation about risks of benzodiazepines *before* tapering. Teach patients relaxation and coping skills *before* you taper benzodiazepines. Go slowly at the beginning of the taper and very slowly at the end when withdrawal symptoms are more likely. Consider mental health consultation for complex patients. Provide patient with educational handouts. Provide individually tailored patient letters with nonpharmacological approaches.

Note. CBT=cognitive-behavioral therapy; D_2=dopamine type 2; IPSRT=interpersonal social rhythm therapy; SNRI=serotonin-norepinephrine reuptake inhibitor; SSRI=selective serotonin reuptake inhibitor.
Source. American Geriatrics Society Expert Panel on Postoperative Delirium in Older Adults 2015; Darker et al. 2015; Jacobson 2014; Tannenbaum et al. 2014.

BASIC PRINCIPLES FOR PREVENTING POLYPHARMACY AND DISCONTINUING PSYCHOTROPIC MEDICATIONS

Always obtain accurate medication lists from each patient or from a caregiver (e.g., in assisted living or skilled nursing facility) and other practitioners.

Ask patients and their caregivers to contact you with updated medication lists after emergency department visits or hospitalizations.

If an adverse effect from a medication is suspected, stop or taper the medication as quickly as possible.

When stopping a medication to simplify a drug regimen, taper it very slowly (weeks to months). It may take weeks to months before patients experience a relapse of their mental health symptoms on a lower dose.

Recording Adverse Medication Effects

Older adults may experience adverse effects from medications prescribed for the treatment of mental disorders. Direction on how to record this information in the medical record is provided in the DSM-5 section "Medication-Induced Movement Disorders and Other Adverse Effects of Medication" (American Psychiatric Association 2013, pp. 709–714). We include Table 16–9 as a summary list from that DSM-5 section so that you can record a movement disorder or other adverse medication effect that is a focus of clinical attention or that may otherwise affect the diagnosis, course, prognosis, or treatment of a patient's mental disorder. A condition listed in the table may be coded if it is a reason for the current visit or helps to explain the need for a test, procedure, or treatment. Conditions and problems from this list also may be included in the medical record as useful information that may affect the patient's care, regardless of relevance to the current visit.

TABLE 16–9. ICD-10-CM codes for adverse medication effects

ICD-10-CM code	Disorder, condition, or problem
G21.11	Neuroleptic-induced parkinsonism
G21.19	Other medication-induced parkinsonism
G21.0	Neuroleptic malignant syndrome
G24.02	Medication-induced acute dystonia
G25.71	Medication-induced acute akathisia
G24.01	Tardive dyskinesia
G24.09	Tardive dystonia
G25.71	Tardive akathisia
G25.1	Medication-induced postural tremor
G25.79	Other medication-induced movement disorder
T43.205A	Antidepressant discontinuation syndrome: initial encounter
T43.205D	Antidepressant discontinuation syndrome: subsequent encounter
T43.205S	Antidepressant discontinuation syndrome: sequelae
T50.905A	Other adverse effect of medication: initial encounter
T50.905D	Other adverse effect of medication: subsequent encounter
T50.905S	Other adverse effect of medication: sequelae

Source. American Psychiatric Association 2013.

CHAPTER 17

Brain Stimulation Therapies

WHEN an older patient fails to respond to other interventions, you should consider treatments that electrically stimulate the brain, either through the direct application of electricity or by the generation of electrical currents with magnets. The most commonly used brain stimulation intervention, electroconvulsive therapy (ECT), can have startling benefits for older patients. ECT is underutilized in community settings, however, both because of stigma around the treatment and because it requires additional resources, including specialized training and equipment; thorough and frequent evaluations; and transportation to and from the procedure. Although these barriers prevent ECT and related treatments from being offered outside of mental health specialty settings at present, these treatments are so essential to geriatric psychiatry that every practitioner needs to be aware of their benefits and risks. The field of brain stimulation interventions is rapidly growing in importance as newer and more convenient techniques are being created.

Electroconvulsive Therapy

Siegfried is an 89-year-old man who is brought to your clinic by his two grandchildren. They are concerned because over the past few months, Siegfried has had significant decreased oral intake and is lying in bed all day. He has lost interest in his family and his hobbies. He appears dysphoric and speaks slowly. Siegfried explains that he is eating less because he has abdominal pain that he believes is due to stomach cancer, although his medical workup for abdominal pain has been negative. You take his blood pressure and realize that he is orthostatic. You admit him to the medical unit and request psychiatry consultation for ECT to treat his probable major depressive disorder with psychotic features.

ECT is one of the oldest and most effective treatments in psychiatry. It is used mainly to treat major depressive disorder, but other indications include mania and Parkinson's disease (Cumper et al. 2014; Medda et al. 2014). ECT works by inducing a generalized tonic-clonic seizure via electrical stimulation delivered through electrodes attached to a patient's scalp. The placement of these electrodes requires a balancing act between maximizing the therapeutic effect and minimizing any adverse effect on cognition. Shorter pulse widths of electrical current are generally used because they are less likely to cause cognitive damage without significantly affecting therapeutic efficacy. One of the most common approaches in ECT is the right unilateral ultrabrief pulse, which maximizes therapeutic efficacy while minimizing adverse cognitive effects (Mankad et al. 2010). No matter what type of ECT is administered, patients undergo anesthesia and are given muscle relaxants to avoid being injured secondary to the induced convulsions (Adachi et al. 2006).

Although ECT can be a quick intervention to help ease suffering from treatment-refractory depression or major depressive disorder with psychosis in older adults, many patients do not pursue this treatment because ECT practitioners are scarce, especially in rural and underserved areas, and finding a caregiver to provide regular transportation to and from the treatment, as often as thrice weekly, may be difficult. Another factor is the negative perception of ECT based on mass media depictions of "shock therapy" when the procedure was still being developed. If primary care or mental health practitioners refer patients for ECT evaluations, they should explain to their patients that today's ECT is a safe, highly standardized procedure that occurs under anesthesia. Practitioners should also inform patients that ECT is highly efficacious, particularly for patients who have not responded to psychotropic medications and psychotherapy (Lisanby 2007). Older adults may particularly benefit from ECT because they are more likely than younger adults to have treatment-refractory depression (Riva-Posse et al. 2013).

ECT, however, does have some significant adverse effects. The most serious are cardiac arrhythmias and other cardiovascular complications. Cardiac clearance for older adults or patients with preexisting cardiac disease is important in order to prevent these complications. It is usually recommended that patients age 50 and older undergo a baseline electrocardiogram (Sundsted et al. 2014). With proper consultation from cardiology and management by anesthesiology, most patients with cardiac disease are still able to receive ECT. The rate of all cardiac complications is 0.9% (Sundsted et al. 2014). Most of these cardiac complications are due to arrhythmias.

Cognitive impairment after ECT is a well-publicized side effect, but large-scale prevalence studies have not been done (Verwijk et al. 2012). It is estimated that cognitive impairment may affect up to 50% of patients, but amnesia is a less frequent problem than it used to be because many practitioners have now modified their procedures to use brief pulse unilateral or ultrabrief pulse ECT to minimize cognitive side effects instead of starting with bilateral ECT (Verwijk et al. 2012). The types of cognitive impairment associated with ECT are anterograde and retrograde amnesia. Generally, anterograde amnesia resolves within a month, whereas retrograde amnesia takes longer to resolve and may not resolve fully, especially in patients who receive ongoing ECT treatments (Lisanby 2007; McClintock et al. 2014; Semkovska and McLoughlin 2010). Some patients' depressive symptoms may not respond to unilateral ECT and may require bilateral ECT; these patients are at much higher risk for cognitive impairment. Another side effect of ECT is postictal delirium, which occurs in about 12% of patients (Fink 1993). Episodes of delirium usually happen with the initial treatments and self-resolve within an hour.

> Siegfried is placed on intravenous fluids and consents to have 10 sessions of ECT to determine whether he will respond. By the fourth session, Siegfried is drinking enough that he no longer requires intravenous fluids. By the tenth session, his delusion that he has stomach cancer and cannot eat is significantly less intense, and his solid intake improves significantly. Siegfried is medically stable enough that he is transferred to inpatient psychiatry to continue his course of ECT, which is given three times a week.
>
> After Siegfried has received ECT for 1 month, he and his grandchildren agree to the recommendation that he have maintenance ECT. After several more months, the maintenance ECT is tapered, and Siegfried maintains fairly good control of his depressive symptoms.

Transcranial Magnetic Stimulation

Transcranial magnetic stimulation (TMS) is another type of brain stimulation therapy. It uses a powerful but brief magnetic field to generate electrical currents within the neurons that have resting potentials, but no currents occur within the rest of the skull and soft tissue. Unlike ECT, TMS does not require electrodes or sedation. In 2008, the U.S. Food and Drug Administration (FDA) approved the NeuroStar TMS Therapy system for treatment of major depressive disorder (Derstine et al. 2010). Several studies have demonstrated the efficacy of TMS as monotherapy and have shown that it has at least similar efficacy as most FDA-approved depressive disorder treatments (George 2010; Janicak et al. 2010; O'Reardon et al. 2007). Studies are under way to determine whether TMS may have use in other psychiatric disorders, such as schizophrenia, obsessive-compulsive disorder (OCD), and posttraumatic stress disorder.

Deep Brain Stimulation

Anita is a 63-year-old woman with treatment-refractory OCD and well-controlled hypertension who complains of worsening compulsions, including excessive hand washing and checking the house for at least 1 hour every day to make sure the doors are locked before she goes out. She spends most of her days inside her home because of fear of contamination from germs in public areas. Anita has already had therapeutic trials of sertraline, fluoxetine, and paroxetine for 3–6 months each. She has also briefly trialed clomipramine, clonazepam, and quetiapine for 2 months each, with only modest improvement on her Yale-Brown Obsessive Compulsive Scale (Y-BOCS) score. Two years ago, Anita spent 6 months at a residential treatment center, where she participated in intensive cognitive-behavioral therapy and exposure and response prevention. You decide to refer her to a specialized psychiatrist who can evaluate her for deep brain stimulation (DBS) to address treatment-refractory OCD.

The consulting psychiatrist concludes that Anita does have treatment-refractory OCD and recommends that she consider DBS to help with her symptoms. Anita consents to the procedure after being informed of the major risks of the surgery, including infection and bleeding. Her Y-BOCS score drops from 38 prior to DBS to 15 after DBS implementation.

DBS was originally developed to treat motor symptoms, including essential tremor, dystonia, and most notably Parkinson's disease (Fasano and Lozano 2015; Okun 2014). The procedure consists of placing an electrode in a targeted area, such as the thalamus, subthalamic nucleus, or globus pallidus. An insulated wire (referred to as "the extension") passes through the skin, head, neck, and shoulder to connect the electrode to a battery-powered pulse generator that is usually implanted underneath the skin near the collarbone or lower chest. Generally, DBS is a well-tolerated procedure; the main postsurgical complications are infection (in 1.7% of patients) and bleeding (in 5%) (Fenoy and Simpson 2014; Hariz 2002). Subthalamic nucleus DBS can also have neuropsychiatric effects. Possible acute effects include euphoria, disinhibition, hyperactivity, hypomania, mania, and impulsive behaviors such as hypersexuality, kleptomania, or intermittent explosive behavior. After implementation, DBS provides a continuous stimulus, whose frequency is customized for each patient, and chronic effects include worsening of depression (which may be confounded by the withdrawal of dopaminergic-inducing drugs after DBS is completed), apathy, improvement of anxiety, and worsening of verbal fluency (most likely from the surgery) and executive functioning (Castrioto et al. 2014).

DBS has a humanitarian device exemption for severe OCD and is being studied for a wide range of psychiatric disorders ranging from treatment-refractory depression to eating disorders. The use of DBS for OCD, however, has not been demonstrated specifically in the geriatric population.

Other Types of Brain Stimulation Interventions

Other types of brain stimulation interventions are still under development or are approved treatments only for carefully selected populations. Vagal nerve stimulation (VNS) is similar to DBS except that the electrical impulses stimulate the vagus nerve instead of the targeted area of the brain. The vagus nerve, also known as cranial nerve X, receives both input and output from various organs throughout the body. VNS was originally developed for partial-onset epilepsy and then was approved by the FDA in 2005 for treatment-refractory depression. It is used infrequently for depression, however, because, despite its approval, questions arose about the rigor of the evidence submitted for the FDA's approval (O'Reardon et al. 2006).

Despite the promise of innovative brain stimulation techniques, large-scale clinical research trials are still needed to answer many questions. Specifically, what are the long-term safety, risks, and efficacy of these treatments? Are other treatments comparable to ECT, which still has the best evidence base of any brain stimulation intervention? Can brain stimulation treatment be used alone, or are the treatments more effective in conjunction with psychopharmacological and/or psychotherapy treatments? We await further innovation and evidence.

CHAPTER 18

Mental Health Treatment Planning

TREATMENT plans can be understood as a regulatory requirement, one of the many chores of contemporary health care, or they can be understood as recipes for changing a patient's life. The goal of any medical intervention is to help a person achieve a therapeutic change he cannot make on his own, and a treatment plan is intended to specify what the person needs to change, who will help him, and how he will make the change. Any reasonable treatment plan will include a problem list, a list of measurable goals, and a recipe for how to achieve those goals.

The reality, of course, is that managing a treatment plan is like both following a recipe and undertaking a chore. The mental health care regulatory requirements of governmental agencies and third-party payers often demand that mental health treatment plans be completed in a proprietary format. Given that reality, we encourage you to identify treatment plans specific to your clinical setting to fulfill the chore aspect but tinker with them like a recipe. In this chapter, we discuss three general principles universal to the recipe aspect of treatment plans: problem lists, patient and caregiver goals, and best practices. They are the what, the who, and the how of treatment plans.

Problem Lists

When you evaluate a person in mental distress, your goal should be to create a therapeutic alliance, but the tangible result of an evaluation is a diagnosis. This diagnosis is the foundation of a treatment plan.

In earlier versions of DSM, diagnoses were described in a multiaxial, or five-axis, system. Practitioners broke a diagnosis into five components: mental illnesses, personality disorders, general medical conditions, psychosocial problems, and global functioning. At its best, the multiaxial system encouraged practitioners to understand a person's distress from multiple perspectives: a biological account of mental illness, a psychological account of personality, a mechanistic account of physical illness, a subjective list of psychosocial factors, and a standardized assessment of functioning. At its worst, the multiaxial system reinforced divisions between mind and body; allowed personality disorders to be used as pejorative slurs; included inconsistent accounts of psychosocial functioning; and jumbled together categories, lists, and assessments. It turned out to be a messy recipe.

The authors of DSM-5 (American Psychiatric Association 2013) reorganized the multiaxial system into a problem list. For physicians, the problem list is familiar because it is already in use throughout medicine. Nonphysicians, however, may benefit from a brief introduction to the problem list. Simply put, a problem list is a comprehensive and hierarchical catalog of the problems addressed during a current encounter.

To benefit communication, the items on the list should be standardized. There are many ways to account for mental distress and mental illness. Individual practitioners may focus on dysfunctional neural circuits, traumatic experiences, or maladaptive personality traits. When these practitioners wish to speak with each other, they need a standard list. The standard list we favor is DSM-5 because it is the consensus diagnostic system of contemporary psychiatry, our way for mental health practitioners to work together while we await a diagnostic system with greater validity.

One reminder that we are awaiting a diagnostic system with improved validity is that the diagnoses generated by a DSM-5 interview are called disorders rather than diseases or illnesses. Physicians usually think in terms of *diseases*, which can be described as pathological abnormalities in the structure and function of body organs and systems. Patients usually present with *illnesses*, their experience of pathological abnormalities or of being sick. From a distance, diseases and illnesses may seem like the same experience viewed from the different perspectives of patient and physician. However, diseases and illnesses are often divergent experiences, not just different perspectives, as anthropologists have repeatedly documented (Estroff and Henderson 2005).

Disorders are a kind of middle path between disease and illness. The term *disorder* acknowledges the complex interplay of biological, social, cultural, and psychological factors in mental distress. Broadly speaking, a disorder simply indicates a disturbance in physical or psychological functioning. Use of the disorder label to describe mental distress draws attention to how mental distress impairs a person's functioning, suggests the complex interplay of events that result in mental distress, and implicitly acknowledges the limits of our knowledge about the causes of mental distress (Kendler 2012). Practitioners in the field do not yet know enough to be more precise. We accept the ongoing use of *disorder* in our diagnostic systems as an opportunity for humility and a spur to further study but primarily as a way to communicate together.

For DSM-5 to work as a common language, practitioners need to agree on the features of a specific diagnosis. Standardization does not work without specificity. Imagine a recipe that lists "a serving of fat" as an ingredient. Someone following the recipe would be confused. Did the author of the recipe mean a spoonful of bacon drippings or a half cup of coconut oil? Each is possible, but each results in a different dish; the recipe becomes more of a personal inspiration than a communal instruction. Similarly, practitioners should recognize that characterizing a person as having "an unspecified mental disorder" inadequately communicates the precise nature of the patient's illness to other practitioners.

We encourage practitioners to select the most specific diagnosis for which a patient qualifies. If you believe a grandmother is depressed, determine not only whether her depression constitutes a major depressive episode but also whether it is a single or recurrent episode, with or without psychotic features, and whether it is mild, moderate, or severe. This level of specificity enables communication with other practitioners and informs their treatment. For example, although we recognize that an adult with a mild first depressive episode would be treated differently from an adult with a severe recurrent depressive episode with psychotic features, we would have trouble deciding how to proceed with an adult diagnosed with a nonspecific mental disorder. Identifying a specific disorder improves communication with a patient's other practitioners while also communicating to the patient and his caregivers your diagnostic ability and understanding of his particular illness. Diagnosis is, itself, a response to a patient's suffering, because giving a specific name to the seemingly unnameable is salutary. (Diagnosis also improves communication with regulators and third-party payers, who frequently reimburse better for more specific diagnoses.)

Sometimes, however, a specific diagnosis is inappropriate. When you are uncertain or need additional information, a provisional diagnosis is always preferable to a specific but inaccurate one. The goal is to eventually arrive at the most specific diagnosis possible. It is discouraging to review medical records in which a person's diagnosis has remained poorly characterized for years.

Even if your diagnoses lack specificity, you can make them comprehensive. They should include all problems—mental disorders, general medical conditions, and psychosocial problems—that are currently diminishing a person's ability to function. As you know by now, we use DSM-5 to describe mental disorders, including the adverse effects from psychiatric treatment, as described in Section II of DSM-5. You also need to describe general medical conditions that currently affect a person's function. You do not need to list well-healed injuries. To describe psychosocial problems that influence a person's health, we favor using the standardized list of ICD-10 codes. Some of the most relevant Z codes are found in Chapter 12, "Rating Scales and Alternative Diagnostic Systems," but the complete list of Z codes, numbered Z00–Z99, is found in the ICD chapter called "Factors Influencing Health Status and Contact With Health Services," which can be found online at http://www.cms.gov/Medicare/coding/ICD10/2016-ICD-10-CM-and-GEMs.html.

Finally, the patient's mental disorders, general medical conditions, and psychosocial problems should be ordered hierarchically. Those problems that are the focus of your treatment at a specific time should lead the list. For example, an older adult may have hypertension, but if you are treating him for an episode of major depressive disorder following an intentional overdose, then his first two problems are his major depressive disorder and his suicide attempt. If you evaluate him again 2 months later and he has recovered from his ingestion and his depressive symptoms are decreased, then his depressive episode and suicide attempt would be lower on the problem list. A well-ordered problem list communicates the focus of your treatment to everyone who reviews your record.

Patient and Caregiver Goals

You develop the goals of treatment through conversation with your patient and his caregivers. Sometimes practitioners ask about goals toward the end of a clinical conversation. We prefer to ask about goals from the beginning and then throughout a conversation. Asking about goals is another way to establish a therapeutic alliance, the mutual commitment you and a patient make to improve his well-being. You and the patient establish the alliance when a patient identifies treatment goals and you ally yourself with him in pursuit of those goals. By doing this early in your encounter, you invariably increase the amount and reliability of information a patient offers. More profoundly, you help motivate a patient's desire to change. We ask, often very directly, "What is your treatment goal?" Then, as the encounter progresses, we frequently check on additional goals, saying something like, "I hear that you are concerned; should we address that as a treatment goal?" By continuing to ask about treatment goals, you clarify the focus of treatment and further build your alliance with a patient.

By the end of a conversation in which you have frequently asked about treatment goals, it is usually straightforward to summarize the most pressing treatment goals. We often do so by saying, "It sounds like we have identified the most important treatment goals, but I want to be certain. Have we identified the right goals?" These kinds of conversations ensure that your treatment goals will reflect a patient's desires, which usually increases his interest in pursuing the treatment goals. When possible and appropriate, you should phrase the treatment goals using the patient's own words.

Part of the challenge of working with older adults with mental distress is bringing patients and caregivers together in pursuit of common goals. With patients, we prefer to identify goals early in an encounter. With caregivers, we like to understand the relationship between a caregiver and a patient before asking about treatment goals. Different caregivers will be invested in a patient in different ways. The caregiver's relationship with the patient—as a spouse, sibling, child, neighbor, religious authority, guardian, or home health aide—affects the treatment goals the caregiver identifies and his ability to effect those goals. You need to know how and why a caregiver is involved in a person's life when soliciting a caregiver's treatment goals.

Once the patient, caregiver, and practitioner agree on treatment goals, it helps the practitioner to consider the settings in which the goals will be pursued. If the problems you mutually identify occur mostly at home, then the goals should focus on the home. If the problems occur mostly at a facility, such as a nursing home, then your goals need to engage the facility's staff and other clients. If you are seeing the patient in a primary care clinic, the treatment goal may include learning coping skills, developing new habits, or establishing care with a mental health practitioner. If you are seeing the patient in a hospital, the treatment goals usually address acute concerns, such as decreasing suicidality or improving mood.

Well-designed treatment goals can help both the practitioner and the patient feel a sense of accomplishment. Setting up realistic, achievable goals requires commitment from the patient and caregiver that they value these goals and will work with you to achieve them. The practitioner should also take into account the patient's age, functional ability, and physical and psychological characteristics, which are important in setting realistic expectations about what can be achieved during a given time period. The treatment goals you set with patients should also be measurable, so you can know whether or not the patient is achieving the goals you have agreed on, and should include a time frame in which they will be completed. For example, instead of telling your patients to "be more physically active," you should set a specific, personal, and measurable goal for a designated time period, such as "Take your dog for a 10-minute walk three times a day for the next 3 months," and then have them keep a journal to record their daily successes.

Best Practices

The medical literature can help in determining what might be achievable and measurable goals for a patient. Although a number of strong texts are available to guide treatment planning (e.g., Reichenberg and Seligman 2016), few resources are available specifically for mental illness treatment planning for older adults. Clinical practice guidelines can often inform a treatment plan. The American Psychiatric Association maintains a set of clinical practice guidelines, which may be found at http://psychiatryonline.org/guidelines; however, these are designed for the treatment of all adult patients, not only older adults. To guide your treatment planning with older adults, we share some general advice for treatment planning in Table 18–1.

TABLE 18–1. Steps in treatment planning for older adults

---

1. Identify your patient's initial treatment goal.

2. Develop a therapeutic alliance with your patient.

3. Clarify the relationship between caregiver(s) and your patient.

4. Reach the most specific DSM-5 diagnosis for your patient.

5. Write a hierarchical, current problem list.

6. Rewrite the problem list into treatment goals.

7. Identify measurable and achievable goals from the available evidence base.

8. Customize the treatment for your patient's cultural background and available resources.

9. Assign responsibility for each goal to a member of your patient's treatment team.

10. Monitor the progress toward each goal.

11. Revise the goals as your patient's situation changes.

CHAPTER 19

Conclusion

The good physician treats the disease, but the great physician treats the patient who has the disease.
—*William Osler*

IN this book, we have discussed common mental health issues that affect older adults, including delirium, major neurocognitive disorder (dementia), depression, drugs causing disorders, sleep disorders (dyssomnias), and mental health symptoms due to medical and neurological disorders. We also have outlined techniques to assess and manage these disorders with a wide range of modalities, including psychopharmacological, psychotherapeutic, and psychosocial.

More than 100 years ago, the renowned neuropathologist Dr. Alois Alzheimer described the neuropsychiatric symptoms of his patient Auguste Deter and identified a disorder that came to be known as Alzheimer's disease. In the early 1900s, discussion of neurodegenerative disorders was limited to monographs and elite academic conferences; however, because the number of older adults affected has increased rapidly, Alzheimer's disease and other geriatric mental disorders have entered the spotlight and transformed society. Despite many scientific advances, the same neuropathology is still being battled, but now on a larger scale.

In 2012, the U.S. National Alzheimer's Project Act (Public Law 111-375) laid out a plan to address the rapidly growing number of adults with Alzheimer's disease and declared the ambitious goal of effectively treating or preventing the disease by 2025 (U.S. Department of Health and Human Services 2016). As the diseases of aging continue to affect society's ability to pay for living and medical expenses of the growing number of older adults, government officials and public policy experts are considering how to restructure Medicare, Social Security, and pension plans. The Institute of

Medicine has been exploring how to address the worsening shortage of geriatric mental health specialists. Currently, there is only one geriatric psychiatrist for approximately every 11,500 Americans, and by 2030, there will be only one for every 20,400 Americans (Institute of Medicine 2012). Researchers and technology companies are pushing various mobile health initiatives to track healthy behaviors, deliver psychotherapies, and create smart home technologies that detect falls and remind individuals to take their pills.

As all of these scientific discoveries, technological advances, and public policy discussions to address the rapidly growing population of older adults are occurring, it is easy to forget that aging is a natural and universal process. Because modern society sees medicine and science as the "fount of youth," taking care of older adults with complex mental, physical, and neurological needs can seem more psychologically challenging than ever.

It is important that you, as a practitioner who bears a portion of the burdens of caring for an aging population with growing mental health needs, strive to make the psychiatric interviewing of older adults a meaningful experience for both you and your patient. DSM-5 (American Psychiatric Association 2013) is a consensus manual developed by experts; our aim was to help you bring their expertise with you to the bedside. To understand the human side of aging, you will learn at the bedside of the people you meet as patients, but you will also learn through art and literature, as well as through relationships with friends and family members who are growing older. We hope you learn from all of these sources and relationships.

References

Acierno R, Hernandez MA, Amstadter AB, et al: Prevalence and correlates of emotional, physical, sexual, and financial abuse and potential neglect in the United States: the National Elder Mistreatment Study. Am J Public Health 100(2):292–297, 2010 20019303

Adachi T, Masumura T, Arai M, et al: Self-administered electroconvulsive treatment with a homemade device. J ECT 22(3):226–227, 2006 16957542

AIMS Center: Care Partners: Bridging Families, Clinics, and Communities to Advance Late-Life Depression Care. 2016. Available at: http://aims.uw.edu/care-partners-bridging-families-clinics-and-communities-advance-late-life-depression-care. Accessed August 18, 2016.

Alexopoulos GS, Raue PJ, Kiosses DN, et al: Problem-solving therapy and supportive therapy in older adults with major depression and executive dysfunction: effect on disability. Arch Gen Psychiatry 68(1):33–41, 2011 21199963

Alzheimer's Association: 2015 Alzheimer's disease facts and figures. Alzheimers Dement 11(3):332–384, 2015a 25984581

Alzheimer's Association: Behaviors: How to Respond When Dementia Causes Unpredictable Behaviors. Chicago, IL, Alzheimer's Association, 2015b. Available at: https://www.alz.org/national/documents/brochure_behaviors.pdf. Accessed August 18, 2016.

Alzheimer's Association: Respite Care. Chicago, IL, Alzheimer's Association, 2016. Available at: https://www.alz.org/care/alzheimers-dementia-caregiver-respite.asp. Accessed August 18, 2016.

American Diabetes Association, American Psychiatric Association, American Association of Clinical Endocrinologists, North American Association for the Study of Obesity: Consensus Development Conference on Antipsychotic Drugs and Obesity and Diabetes. J Clin Psychiatry 65(2):267–272, 2004 15003083

American Foundation for Suicide Prevention: Suicide Statistics. New York, American Foundation for Suicide Prevention, 2015. Available at: https://www.afsp.org/understanding-suicide/facts-and-figures. Accessed August 18, 2016.

American Geriatrics Society Expert Panel on Postoperative Delirium in Older Adults: Postoperative delirium in older adults: best practice statement from the American Geriatrics Society. J Am Coll Surg 220(2):136–148.e1, 2015 25535170

American Occupational Therapy Association: Dementia and the Role of Occupational Therapy. Bethesda, MD, American Occupational Therapy Association, 2016. Available at: http://www.aota.org/about-occupational-therapy/professionals/mh/dementia.aspx. Accessed August 18, 2016.

American Psychiatric Association: Diagnostic and Statistical Manual of Mental Disorders, 3rd Edition. Washington, DC, American Psychiatric Association, 1980

American Psychiatric Association: Diagnostic and Statistical Manual of Mental Disorders, 4th Edition, Text Revision. Washington, DC, American Psychiatric Association, 2000

American Psychiatric Association: Diagnostic and Statistical Manual of Mental Disorders, 5th Edition. Arlington, VA, American Psychiatric Association, 2013

American Psychiatric Association: Major Depressive Disorder and the "Bereavement Exclusion." Arlington, VA, American Psychiatric Association, 2015a. Available at: http://www.dsm5.org/Documents/Bereavement%20Exclusion%20Fact%20Sheet.pdf. Accessed August 18, 2016.

American Psychiatric Association: Understanding Mental Disorders: Your Guide to DSM-5. Arlington, VA, American Psychiatric Association, 2015b

American Psychiatric Association Work Group on Psychiatric Evaluation: The American Psychiatric Association Practice Guidelines for the Psychiatric Evaluation of Adults, 3rd Edition. Arlington, VA, American Psychiatric Association, 2016

American Sleep Association: Hallucinations During Sleep. Lititz, PA, American Sleep Association, September 2007. Available at: https://www.sleepassociation.org/patients-general-public/hallucinations-during-sleep/. Accessed August 18, 2016.

Anderson F, Downing GM, Hill J, et al: Palliative Performance Scale (PPS): a new tool. J Palliat Care 12(1):5–11, 1996 8857241

Asnis GM, Henderson MA: Levomilnacipran for the treatment of major depressive disorder: a review. Neuropsychiatr Dis Treat 11:125–135, 2015 25657584

AstraZeneca: Pharameuticals LP. Seroquel tablets, 2003. Available at http://www.accessdata.fda.gov/drugsatfda_docs/label/2004/20639se1-017,016_seroquel_lbl.pdf. Accessed August 26, 2016.

Aurora RN, Kristo DA, Bista SR, et al: The treatment of restless legs syndrome and periodic limb movement disorder in adults—an update for 2012: practice parameters with an evidence-based systematic review and meta-analyses: an American Academy of Sleep Medicine Clinical Practice Guideline. Sleep 35(8):1039–1062, 2012 22851801

Austin BJ, Fleisher LK: Financing End-of-Life Care: Challenges for an Aging Population. Washington, DC, Academy Health, 2003. Available at: http://www.hcfo.org/pdf/eolcare.pdf. Accessed August 18, 2016.

Bäärnhielm S, Scarpinati Rosso M: The Cultural Formulation: a model to combine nosology and patients' life context in psychiatric diagnostic practice. Transcult Psychiatry 46(3):406–428, 2009 19837779

Babor TF, de la Fuente JR, Saunders JB, Grant M: The Alcohol Use Disorders Identification Test: Guidelines for Use in Primary Health Care. Geneva, World Health Organization, 1989

Bang J, Spina S, Miller BL: Frontotemporal dementia. Lancet 386:1672–1682, 2015 26595641

Bakker R: GEM Environmental Assessment: Gerontological Environmental Modifications. New York, Cornell University, Joan and Sanford I. Weill Medical College, 2005. Available at: http://www.environmentalgeriatrics.com/pdf/enviro_assessment.pdf. Accessed August 18, 2016.

Bankoff SM, Karpel MG, Forbes HE, Pantalone DW: A systematic review of dialectical behavior therapy for the treatment of eating disorders. Eat Disord 20(3):196–215, 2012 22519897

Beck Institute of Cognitive Behavior Therapy: What Is Cognitive Behavior Therapy? Bala Cynwyd, PA, Beck Institute of Cognitive Behavior Therapy, 2016. Available at: https://www.beckinstitute.org/faq/what-is-cognitive-behavior-therapy/. Accessed August 18, 2016.

Bennett T, Bray D, Neville MW: Suvorexant, a dual orexin receptor antagonist for the management of insomnia. P&T 39(4):264–266, 2014 24757363

Benson WF, Aldrich N: Advance Care Planning: Ensuring Your Wishes Are Known and Honored If You Are Unable to Speak for Yourself. Critical Issue Brief. Atlanta, GA, Centers for Disease Control and Prevention, 2012. Available at: http://www.cdc.gov/aging/pdf/advanced-care-planning-critical-issue-brief.pdf. Accessed August 18, 2016.

Berg KO, Wood-Dauphinee SL, Williams JI, Maki B: Measuring balance in the elderly: validation of an instrument. Can J Public Health 83 (suppl 2):S7–S11, 1992 1468055

Berganza CE, Mezzich JE, Jorge MR: Latin American Guide for Psychiatric Diagnosis (GLDP). Psychopathology 35(2–3):185–190, 2002 12145508

Billings JA: The need for safeguards in advance care planning. J Gen Intern Med 27(5):595–600, 2012 22237664

Blais MA, Baer L: Understanding rating scales and assessment instruments, in Handbook of Clinical Rating Scales and Assessment in Psychiatry and Mental Health (Current Clinical Psychiatry). Edited by Baer L, Blais MA. New York, Humana Press, 2010, pp 2–6

Blazer DG: Psychiatry and the oldest old. Am J Psychiatry 157(12):1915–1924, 2000 11097951

Blow FC, Brower KJ, Schulenberg JE, et al: The Michigan Alcoholism Screening Test–Geriatric Version (MAST-G): a new elderly-specific screening instrument. Alcohol Clin Exp Res 16:372–374, 1992

Bruce ML, Ten Have TR, Reynolds CF III, et al: Reducing suicidal ideation and depressive symptoms in depressed older primary care patients: a randomized controlled trial. JAMA 291(9):1081–1091, 2004 14996777

Buck CJ: ICD-10-CM. St. Louis, MO, Elsevier, 2017

Budnitz DS, Lovegrove MC, Shehab N, Richards CL: Emergency hospitalizations for adverse drug events in older Americans. N Engl J Med 365(21):2002–2012, 2011 22111719

Byers AL, Yaffe K: Depression and risk of developing dementia. Nat Rev Neurol 7(6):323–331, 2011 21537355

Carreira K, Miller MD, Frank E, et al: A controlled evaluation of monthly maintenance interpersonal psychotherapy in late-life depression with varying levels of cognitive function. Int J Geriatr Psychiatry 23(11):1110–1113, 2008 18457338

Castrioto A, Lhommée E, Moro E, Krack P: Mood and behavioural effects of subthalamic stimulation in Parkinson's disease. Lancet Neurol 13(3):287–305, 2014 24556007

Catalán R, Penadés R: Risperidone long-acting injection: safety and efficacy in elderly patients with schizophrenia. J Cent Nerv Syst Dis 3:95–105, 2011 23861642

Centers for Disease Control and Prevention: Check for Safety: A Home Fall Prevention Checklist for Older Adults. 2015. Available at: http://www.cdc.gov/steadi/pdf/check_for_safety_brochure-a.pdf. Accessed August 18, 2016

Centers for Disease Control and Prevention: Important facts about falls, January 2016. Available at: www.cdc.gov/homeandrecreational safety/falls/adultfalls.html. Accessed August 25, 2016.

Chen YF: Chinese classification of mental disorders (CCMD-3): towards integration in international classification. Psychopathology 35(2–3):171–175, 2002 12145505

Clozapine REMS Program: Recommended Monitoring Frequency and Clinical Decisions by ANC Level. Phoenix, AZ, Clozapine REMS Program, 2014. Available at: https://www.clozapinerems.com/CpmgClozapineUI/rems/pdf/resources/ANC_Table.pdf. Accessed August 18, 2016.

Collin C, Wade DT, Davies S, Horne V: The Barthel ADL Index: a reliability study. Int Disabil Stud 10(2):61–63, 1988 3403500

Collins LG, Swartz K: Caregiver care. Am Fam Physician 83(11):1309–1317, 2011 21661713

Conway KP, Compton W, Stinson FS, Grant BF: Lifetime comorbidity of DSM-IV mood and anxiety disorders and specific drug use disorders: results from the National Epidemiologic Survey on Alcohol and Related Conditions. J Clin Psychiatry 67(2):247–257, 2006 16566620

Croft HA, Pomara N, Gommoll C, et al: Efficacy and safety of vilazodone in major depressive disorder: a randomized, double-blind, placebo-controlled trial. J Clin Psychiatry 75(11):e1291–e1298, 2014 25470094

Cullison SK, Resch WJ, Thomas CJ: How should you use the lab to monitor patients taking a mood stabilizer? Curr Psychiatr 13(7):51–55, 2014

Cummings JL, Mega M, Gray K, et al: The Neuropsychiatric Inventory: comprehensive assessment of psychopathology in dementia. Neurology 44(12):2308–2314, 1994 7991117

Cumper SK, Ahle GM, Liebman LS, Kellner CH: Electroconvulsive therapy (ECT) in Parkinson's disease: ECS and dopamine enhancement. J ECT 30(2):122–124, 2014 24810775

Darker CD, Sweeney BP, Barry JM, et al: Psychosocial interventions for benzodiazepine harmful use, abuse or dependence. Cochrane Database Syst Rev 5:CD009652, 2015 26114884

Davidson J: Seizures and bupropion: a review. J Clin Psychiatry 50(7):256–261, 1989 2500425

Depp CA, Lebowitz BD, Patterson TL, et al: Medication adherence skills training for middle-aged and elderly adults with bipolar disorder: development and pilot study. Bipolar Disord 9(6):636–645, 2007 17845279

Derstine T, Lanocha K, Wahlstrom C, Hutton TM: Transcranial magnetic stimulation for major depressive disorder: a pragmatic approach to implementing TMS in a clinical practice. Ann Clin Psychiatry 22(4 suppl):S4–S11, 2010 21180663

Dobkin RD, Menza M, Allen LA, et al: Cognitive-behavioral therapy for depression in Parkinson's disease: a randomized, controlled trial. Am J Psychiatry 168(10):1066–1074, 2011 21676990

Dubois B, Slachevsky A, Litvan I, Pillon B: The FAB: a Frontal Assessment Battery at bedside. Neurology 55(11):1621–1626, 2000 11113214

Emanuel EJ, Emanuel LL: Four models of the physician-patient relationship. JAMA 267(16):2221–2226, 1992 1556799

Epping EA, Kim JI, Craufurd D, et al: Longitudinal psychiatric symptoms in prodromal Huntington's disease: a decade of data. Am J Psychiatry 173(2):184–192, 2016 26472629

Estroff SE, Henderson GE: Social and cultural contributions to health, difference, and inequality, in The Social Medicine Reader, 2nd Edition, Vol 2. Durham, NC, Duke University Press, 2005, pp 4–26

Fasano A, Lozano AM: Deep brain stimulation for movement disorders: 2015 and beyond. Curr Opin Neurol 28(4):423–436, 2015 26110808

Feder J, Komisar H: The Importance of Federal Financing to the Nation's Long-Term Care Safety Net. Long Beach, CA, The SCAN Foundation, February 2012, p 3. Available at: http://www.thescanfoundation.org/importance-federal-financing-nations-long-term-care-safety-net. Accessed August 18, 2016.

Feinstein AR: Clinical Judgment. Baltimore, MD, Williams & Wilkins, 1967

Fenoy AJ, Simpson RK Jr: Risks of common complications in deep brain stimulation surgery: management and avoidance. J Neurosurg 120(1):132–139, 2014 24236657

Fink A, Morton SC, Beck JC, et al: The Alcohol-Related Problems Survey: identifying hazardous and harmful drinking in older primary care patients. J Am Geriatr Soc 50(10):1717–1722, 2002 12366628

Fink M: Post-ECT delirium. Convuls Ther 9(4):326–330, 1993 11941228

First MB: DSM-5 Handbook of Differential Diagnosis. Washington, DC, American Psychiatric Publishing, 2014

Folstein MF, Folstein SE, McHugh PR: "Mini-mental state": a practical method for grading the cognitive state of patients for the clinician. J Psychiatr Res 12(3):189–198, 1975 1202204

Forsaa EB, Larsen JP, Wentzel-Larsen T, et al: A 12-year population-based study of psychosis in Parkinson disease. Arch Neurol 67(8):996–1001, 2010 20697051

Forester B, Sajatovic M, Tsai J, et al: Long-term treatment with lurasidone in older adults with bipolar depression: results of a 6 month open-label study. Eur Psychiatry 30 (suppl 1):23–31, 2015

Fournier JC, DeRubeis RJ, Hollon SD, et al: Antidepressant drug effects and depression severity: a patient-level meta-analysis. JAMA 303(1):47–53, 2010 20051569

Francis JL, Kumar A: Psychological treatment of late-life depression. Psychiatr Clin North Am 36(4):561–575, 2013 24229657

Garfinkel D, Mangin D: Feasibility study of a systematic approach for discontinuation of multiple medications in older adults: addressing polypharmacy. Arch Intern Med 170(18):1648–1654, 2010 20937924

George MS: Transcranial magnetic stimulation for the treatment of depression. Expert Rev Neurother 10(11):1761–1772, 2010 20977332

Gitlin LN, Kales HC, Lyketsos CG: Nonpharmacologic management of behavioral symptoms in dementia. JAMA 308(19):2020–2029, 2012 23168825

GlaxoSmithKline: Lamotrigine prescribing 2015 information, 2015. Available at https://gsksource.com/pharma/content/dam/GlaxoSmithKline/US/en/Prescribing_Information/Lamictal/pdf/LAMICTAL-PI-MG.PDF. Accessed August 26, 2016.

Gould RL, Coulson MC, Howard RJ: Cognitive behavioral therapy for depression in older people: a meta-analysis and meta-regression of randomized controlled trials. J Am Geriatr Soc 60(10):1817–1830, 2012 23003115

Greenberger D, Padesky CA: Mind Over Mood: Change How You Feel by Changing the Way You Think, 2nd Edition. New York, Guilford, 2015

Gury C, Cousin F: Pharmacokinetics of SSRI antidepressants: half-life and clinical applicability [in French]. Encephale 25(5):470–476, 1999 10598311

Gustafsson H, Nordström A, Nordström P: Depression and subsequent risk of Parkinson disease: a nationwide cohort study. Neurology 84(24):2422–2429, 2015 25995056

Hariz MI: Complications of deep brain stimulation surgery. Mov Disord 17 (suppl 3):S162–S166, 2002 11948772

Harrington C, Carrillo H, Garfield R: Nursing facilities, staffing, residents and facilty deficiences, 2009 through 2014. Washington, DC, Henry J Kaiser Foundation, 2015. Available at: http://kff.org/medicaid/report/nursing-facilities-staffing-residents-and-facility-deficiencies-2009-through-2014. Accessed August 18, 2016.

Harris-Kojetin L, Sengupta M, Park-Lee E, et al: Long-term care services in the United States: 2013 overview: National Center for Health Statistics. Vital Health Stat 3 (37):1–107, 2013

Harris-Kojetin L, Sengupta M, Park-Lee E, et al: Long-term care providers and services users in the United States: data from the National Study of Long-Term Care Providers, 2013–2014. Vital Health Stat 3 (38):1–118, 2016 27023287

Hatta K, Kishi Y, Wada K, et al: Preventive effects of ramelteon on delirium: a randomized placebo-controlled trial. JAMA Psychiatry 71(4):397–403, 2014 24554232

Heisel MJ, Talbot NL, King DA, et al: Adapting interpersonal psychotherapy for older adults at risk for suicide. Am J Geriatr Psychiatry 23(1):87–98, 2015 24840611

Hickam DH, Weiss JW, Guise J-M, et al: Outpatient Case Management for Adults With Medical Illness and Complex Care Needs (Report No 13-EHC031-EF). Rockville, MD, Agency for Healthcare Research and Quality, January 2013

Hofmann SG, Asnaani A, Vonk IJ, et al: The efficacy of cognitive behavoral therapy: a review of meta-analyses. Cognit Ther Res 26(5):427–440, 2012 23459093

Hogan C, Lunney J, Gabel J, Lynn J: Medicare beneficiaries' costs of care in the last year of life. Health Aff (Millwood) 20(4):188–195, 2001 11463076

Holmes TH, Rahe RH: The Social Readjustment Rating Scale. J Psychosom Res 11(2):213–218, 1967 6059863

Holt AEM, Albert ML: Cognitive neuroscience of delusions in aging. Neuropsychiatr Dis Treat 2(11):181–189, 2006 19412462

Inouye SK: Delirium in older persons. N Engl J Med 354(11):1157–1165, 2006 16540616

Inouye SK, van Dyck CH, Alessi CA, et al: Clarifying confusion: the Confusion Assessment Method: a new method for detection of delirium. Ann Intern Med 113(12):941–948, 1990 2240918

Insel T, Cuthbert B, Garvey M, et al: Research Domain Criteria (RDoC): toward a new classification framework for research on mental disorders. Am J Psychiatry 167(7):748–751, 2010 20595427

Institute of Medicine: The Mental Health and Substance Use Workforce for Older Adults: In Whose Hands? Washington, DC, National Academies Press, 2012

Jacobson SA: Clinical Manual of Geriatric Psychopharmacology, 2nd Edition. Arlington, VA, American Psychiatric Publishing, 2014

Janicak PG, Nahas Z, Lisanby SH, et al: Durability of clinical benefit with transcranial magnetic stimulation (TMS) in the treatment of pharmacoresistant major depression: assessment of relapse during a 6-month, multisite, open-label study. Brain Stimul 3(4):187–199, 2010 20965447

Jones AL, Moss AJ, Harris-Kojetin LD: Use of Advance Directives in Long-Term Care Populations (NCHS Data Brief No 54). Hyattsville, MD, National Center for Health Statistics, January 2011. Available at: http://www.cdc.gov/nchs/data/databriefs/db54.pdf. Accessed August 18, 2016.

Jorge RE: Mood disorders. Handb Clin Neurol 128:613–631, 2015 25701910

Jorge RE, Robinson RG, Starkstein SE, et al: Secondary mania following traumatic brain injury. Am J Psychiatry 150(6):916–921, 1993 8494069

Kales HC, Gitlin LN, Lyketsos CG, et al: Management of neuropsychiatric symptoms of dementia in clinical settings: recommendations from a multidisciplinary expert panel. J Am Geriatr Soc 62(4):762–769, 2014 24635665

Kasl-Godley JE, Christie KM: Advanced illness and the end of life, in Oxford Handbook of Clinical Geropsychology. Edited by Pachana NA, Laidlaw K. Oxford, UK, Oxford University Press, 2014, pp 355–380

Kass-Bartelmes BL: Advance Care Planning: Preferences for Care at the End of Life. Research in Action Issue 12. Rockville, MD, Agency for Healthcare Research and Quality, March 2003. Available at: http://archive.ahrq.gov/research/findings/factsheets/aging/endliferia/endria.pdf. Accessed August 18, 2016.

Katz S, Ford AB, Moskowitz RW, et al: Studies of illness in the aged. The index of ADL: a standardized measure of biological and psychosocial function. JAMA 185:914–919, 1963 14044222

Kaufman DM, Milstein MJ: Kaufman's Clinical Neurology for Psychiatrists, 7th Edition. New York, WB Saunders/Elsevier, 2013

Kendell R, Jablensky A: Distinguishing between the validity and utility of psychiatric diagnoses. Am J Psychiatry 160(1):4–12, 2003 12505793

Kendler KS: The dappled nature of causes of psychiatric illness: replacing the organic-functional/hardware-software dichotomy with empirically based pluralism. Mol Psychiatry 17(4):377–388, 2012 22230881

Kessel B: Sexuality in the older person. Age Ageing 30(2):121–124, 2001 11395341

Kessler RC, Sonnega A, Bromet E, et al: Posttraumatic stress disorder in the National Comorbidity Survey. Arch Gen Psychiatry 52(12):1048–1060, 1995 7492257

Kinghorn WA: Whose disorder? A constructive MacIntyrean critique of psychiatric nosology. J Med Philos 36(2):187–205, 2011 21357652

Kiosses DN, Alexopoulos GS: Problem-solving therapy in the elderly. Curr Treat Options Psychiatry 1(1):15–26, 2014 24729951

Kiosses DN, Arean PA, Teri L, Alexopoulos GS: Home-delivered problem adaptation therapy (PATH) for depressed, cognitively impaired, disabled elders: a preliminary study. Am J Geriatr Psychiatry 18(11):988–998, 2010 20808092

Kroenke K, Spitzer RL, Williams JB: The PHQ-9: validity of a brief depression severity measure. J Gen Intern Med 16(9):606–613, 2001 11556941

Kunik ME, Braun U, Stanley MA, et al: One session cognitive behavioural therapy for elderly patients with chronic obstructive pulmonary disease. Psychol Med 31(4):717–723, 2001 11352373

LaMantia MA, Alder CA, Callahan CM, et al: The Aging Brain Care Medical Home: preliminary data. J Am Geriatr Soc 63(6):1209–1213, 2015 26096394

Lanata SC, Miller BL: The behavioural variant frontotemporal dementia (bvFTD) syndrome in psychiatry. J Neurol Neurosurg Psychiatry 87(5):501–511, 2016 26216940

Laughren TP, Gobburu J, Temple RJ, et al: Vilazodone: clinical basis for the U.S. Food and Drug Administration's approval of a new antidepressant. J Clin Psychiatry 72(9):1166–1173, 2011 21951984

Lawton MP, Brody EM: Assessment of older people: self-maintaining and instrumental activities of daily living. Gerontologist 9(3):179–186, 1969 5349366

Lee SJ, Go AS, Lindquist K, et al: Chronic conditions and mortality among the oldest old. Am J Public Health 98(7):1209–1214, 2008 18511714

Lenze EJ, Sheffrin M, Driscoll HC, et al: Incomplete response in late-life depression: getting to remission. Dialogues Clin Neurosci 10(4):419–430, 2008 19170399

Lewis-Fernández R, Aggarwal NK, Hinton L, et al: DSM-5 Handbook on the Cultural Formulation Interview. Arlington, VA, American Psychiatric Publishing, 2015

Lieb K, Zanarini MC, Schmahl C, et al: Borderline personality disorder. Lancet 364(9432):453–461, 2004 15288745

Lim R: Clinical Manual of Cultural Psychiatry, 2nd Edition. Arlington, VA, American Psychiatric Publishing, 2015

Lisanby SH: Electroconvulsive therapy for depression. N Engl J Med 357(19):1939–1945, 2007 17989386

Lizardi D, Oquendo MA, Graver R: Clinical pitfalls in the diagnosis of ataque de nervios: a case study. Transcult Psychiatry 46(3):463–486, 2009 19837782

Llanque SM, Enriquez M, Cheng AL, et al: The Family Series Workshop: a community-based psychoeducational intervention. Am J Alzheimers Dis Other Demen 30(6):573–583, 2015 25609602

Lynch TR: Treatment of elderly depression with personality disorder comorbidity using dialectical behavior therapy. Cogn Behav Pract 7(4):468–477, 2000

Lynch TR, Morse JQ, Mendelson T, Robins CJ: Dialectical behavior therapy for depressed older adults: a randomized pilot study. Am J Geriatr Psychiatry 11(1):33–45, 2003 12527538

Lynch TR, Cheavens JS, Cukrowicz KC, et al: Treatment of older adults with co-morbid personality disorder and depression: a dialectical behavior therapy approach. Int J Geriatr Psychiatry 22(2):131–143, 2007 17096462

MacIntyre AC: Dependent Rational Animals: Why Human Beings Need the Virtues. Chicago, IL, Open Court Publishing, 2012

Mankad MV, Beyer JL, Krystal AD, Weiner RD: Clinical Manual of Electroconvulsive Therapy. Washington, DC, American Psychiatric Publishing, 2010

Marek KD, Antle L: Medication management of the community-dwelling older adult, in Patient Safety and Quality: An Evidence-Based Handbook for Nurses (AHRQ Publ No 08-0043). Edited by Hughes RG. Rockville, MD, Agency for Healthcare Research and Quality, April 2008, pp 1–38. Available at: http://archive.ahrq.gov/professionals/clinicians-providers/resources/nursing/resources/nurseshdbk/nurseshdbk.pdf. Accessed August 18, 2016.

Martín-Carrasco M, Domínguez-Panchón AI, González-Fraile E, et al: Effectiveness of a psychoeducational intervention group program in the reduction of the burden experienced by caregivers of patients with dementia: the EDUCA-II randomized trial. Alzheimer Dis Assoc Disord 28(1):79–87, 2014 24113563

Martínez LC: DSM-IV-TR cultural formulation of psychiatric cases: two proposals for clinicians. Transcult Psychiatry 46(3):506–523, 2009 19837784

Mathias S, Nayak US, Isaacs B: Balance in elderly patients: the "get-up and go" test. Arch Phys Med Rehabil 67(6):387–389, 1986 3487300

McClintock SM, Choi J, Deng ZD, et al: Multifactorial determinants of the neurocognitive effects of electroconvulsive therapy. J ECT 30(2):165–176, 2014 24820942

McCurry SM, Logsdon RG, Teri L, Vitiello MV: Evidence-based psychological treatments for insomnia in older adults. Psychol Aging 22(1):18–27, 2007 17385979

McDowell AK, Lineberry TW, Bostwick JM: Practical suicide-risk management for the busy primary care physician. Mayo Clin Proc 86(8):792–800, 2011 21709131

Medda P, Toni C, Perugi G: The mood-stabilizing effects of electroconvulsive therapy. J ECT 30(4):275–282, 2014 25010031

Medicaid.gov: PACE Benefits. Baltimore, MD, Centers for Medicare & Medicaid Services, 2016a. Available at: http://www.medicaid.gov/medicaid-chip-program-information/by-topics/long-term-services-and-supports/integrating-care/program-of-all-inclusive-care-for-the-elderly-pace/pace-benefits.html. Accessed August 18, 2016.

Medicaid.gov: Program of All-Inclusive Care for the Elderly (PACE). 2016b. Available at: http://www.medicaid.gov/Medicaid-CHIP-Program-Information/By-Topics/Long-Term-Services-and-Supports/Integrating-Care/Program-of-All-Inclusive-Care-for-the-Elderly-PACE/Program-of-All-Inclusive-Care-for-the-Elderly-PACE.html. Accessed August 18, 2016.

Meltzer HY: Update on typical and atypical antipsychotic drugs. Annu Rev Med 65:393–406, 2013 23020880

Menon GJ, Rahman I, Menon SJ, Dutton GN: Complex visual hallucinations in the visually impaired: the Charles Bonnet syndrome. Surv Ophthalmol 48(1):58–72, 2003 12559327

Miller MD, Reynolds CF III: Expanding the usefulness of Interpersonal Psychotherapy (IPT) for depressed elders with co-morbid cognitive impairment. Int J Geriatr Psychiatry 22(2):101–105, 2007 17096459

Mohlman J, Gorenstein EE, Kleber M, et al: Standard and enhanced cognitive-behavior therapy for late-life generalized anxiety disorder: two pilot investigations. Am J Geriatr Psychiatry 11(1):24–32, 2003 12527537

Mol A: The Logic of Care: Health and the Problem of Choice. New York, Routledge, 2008

Morgan AC: Practical geriatrics: psychodynamic psychotherapy with older adults. Psychiatr Serv 54(12):1592–1594, 2003 14645796

Moseley D, Gala G: Philosophy and Psychiatry: Problems, Intersections, and New Perspectives. New York, Routledge, 2015

Muayqil T, Gronseth G, Camicioli R: Evidence-based guideline: diagnostic accuracy of CSF 14-3-3 protein in sporadic Creutzfeldt-Jakob disease: report of the Guideline Development Subcommittee of the American Academy of Neurology. Neurology 79(14):1499–1506, 2012 22993290

Nakane Y, Nakane H: Classification systems for psychiatric diseases currently used in Japan. Psychopathology 35(2–3):191–194, 2002 12145509

Nasreddine ZS, Phillips NA, Bédirian V, et al: The Montreal Cognitive Assessment, MoCA: a brief screening tool for mild cognitive impairment. J Am Geriatr Soc 53(4):695–699, 2005 15817019

National Adult Day Services Association: Overview and facts. 2016. Available at: http://nadsa.org/consumers/overview-and-facts/. Accessed August 18, 2016.

National Institute on Aging: Talking With Your Older Patient: A Clinician's Handbook. Bethesda, MD, National Institute of Mental Health, April 2016. Available at: https://www.nia.nih.gov/health/publication/talking-your-older-patient. Accessed August 24, 2016.

National Institute of Neurological Disorders and Stroke: Restless Legs Syndrome Fact Sheet. Bethesda, MD, National Institute of Neurological Disorders and Stroke, July 2015. Available at: www.ninds.nih.gov/disorders/restless_legs/detail_restless_legs.htm. Accessed August 24, 2016.

Novartis: Tegretol, 2015. Available at https://www.pharma.us.novartis.com/sites/www.pharma.us.novartis.com/files/tegretol.pdf. Accessed August 27, 2016.

Nussbaum AM: Pocket Guide to the DSM-5 Diagnostic Exam. Washington, DC, American Psychiatric Publishing, 2013

Okun MS: Deep-brain stimulation—entering the era of human neural-network modulation. N Engl J Med 371(15):1369–1373, 2014 25197963

O'Reardon JP, Cristancho P, Peshek AD: Vagus nerve stimulation (VNS) and treatment of depression: to the brainstem and beyond. Psychiatry (Edgmont) 3(5):54–63, 2006 21103178

O'Reardon JP, Solvason HB, Janicak PG, et al: Efficacy and safety of transcranial magnetic stimulation in the acute treatment of major depression: a multisite randomized controlled trial. Biol Psychiatry 62(11):1208–1216, 2007 17573044

Otero-Ojeda AA: Third Cuban Glossary of Psychiatry (GC-3): key features and contributions. Psychopathology 35(2–3):181–184, 2002 12145507

Overall JE, Gorham DR: The Brief Psychiatric Rating Scale. Psychol Rep 10:799–812, 1962

Rabins PV, Starkstein SE, Robinson RG: Risk factors for developing atypical (schizophreniform) psychosis following stroke. J Neuropsychiatry Clin Neurosci 3(1):6–9, 1991 7580174

Radden J, Sadler JZ: The Virtuous Psychiatrist: Character Ethics in Psychiatric Practice. New York, Oxford University Press, 2010

Rauch AS, Fleischhacker WW: Long-acting injectable formulations of new-generation antipsychotics: a review from a clinical perspective. CNS Drugs 27(8):637–652, 2013 23780619

Ray WA, Chung CP, Murray KT, et al: Atypical antipsychotic drugs and the risk of sudden cardiac death. N Engl J Med 360(3):225–235, 2009 19144938

Reichenberg LW, Seligman L: Selecting Effective Treatments, 5th Edition. New York, Wiley, 2016

Reynolds CF III, Frank E, Perel JM, et al: Nortriptyline and interpersonal psychotherapy as maintenance therapies for recurrent major depression: a randomized controlled trial in patients older than 59 years. JAMA 281(1):39–45, 1999a 9892449

Reynolds CF III, Miller MD, Pasternak RE, et al: Treatment of bereavement-related major depressive episodes in later life: a controlled study of acute and continuation treatment with nortriptyline and interpersonal psychotherapy. Am J Psychiatry 156(2):202–208, 1999b 9989555

Reynolds CF III, Dew MA, Pollock BG, et al: Maintenance treatment of major depression in old age. N Engl J Med 354(11):1130–1138, 2006 16540613

Reynolds CF III, Dew MA, Martire LM, et al: Treating depression to remission in older adults: a controlled evaluation of combined escitalopram with interpersonal psychotherapy versus escitalopram with depression care management. Int J Geriatr Psychiatry 25(11):1134–1141, 2010 20957693

Riva-Posse P, Hermida AP, McDonald WM: The role of electroconvulsive and neuromodulation therapies in the treatment of geriatric depression. Psychiatr Clin North Am 36(4):607–630, 2013 24229660

Rojas-Fernandez CH, Chen Y: Use of ultra-low-dose (≤6 mg) doxepin for treatment of insomnia in older people. Can Pharm J (Ott) 147(5):281–289, 2014 25364337

Roseborough DJ, Luptak M, McLeod J, Bradshaw W: Effectiveness of psychodynamic psychotherapy with older adults: a longitudinal study. Clin Gerontol 36(1):1–16, 2013

Rosenblatt A: Neuropsychiatry of Huntington's disease. Dialogues Clin Neurosci 9(2):191–197, 2007 17726917

Roth T: Insomnia: definition, prevalence, etiology, and consequences. J Clin Sleep Med 3(5)(suppl):S7–S10, 2007 17824495

Royall DR, Mahurin RK, Gray KF: Bedside assessment of executive cognitive impairment: the Executive Interview. J Am Geriatr Soc 40(12):1221–1226, 1992 1447438

Sajatovic M, Forester BP, Tsai J, et al: Efficacy of lurasidone in adults aged 55 years and older with bipolar depression: post hoc analysis of 2 double-blind, placebo-controlled studies. J Clin Psychiatry Aug 16, 2016 [Epub ahead of print] 27529375

Salzman C: Clinical Geriatric Psychopharmacology, 4th Edition. Philadelphia, PA, Lippincott Williams & Wilkins, 2005

Santos CO, Caeiro L, Ferro JM, Figueira ML: Mania and stroke: a systematic review. Cerebrovasc Dis 32(1):11–21, 2011 21576938

Scheidemantel T, Korobkova I, Rej S, Sajatovic M: Asenapine for bipolar disorder. Neuropsychiatr Dis Treat 11:3007–3017, 2015 26674884

Schering Corporation: Trilafin tablets and trilafon injection, 2002. Available at http://www.accessdata.fda.gov/drugsatfda_docs/label/2002/10775s311213s24lbl.pdf. Accessed August 27, 2016.

Semkovska M, McLoughlin DM: Objective cognitive performance associated with electroconvulsive therapy for depression: a systematic review and meta-analysis. Biol Psychiatry 68(6):568–577, 2010 20673880

Shahrokh NC, Hales RE, Phillips KA, et al: The Language of Mental Health: A Glossary of Psychiatric Terms. Washington, DC, American Psychiatric Publishing, 2011

Sherrill JT, Frank E, Geary M, et al: Psychoeducational workshops for elderly patients with recurrent major depression and their families. Psychiatr Serv 48(1):76–81, 1997 9117505

Shukla S, Cook BL, Mukherjee S, et al: Mania following head trauma. Am J Psychiatry 144(1):93–96, 1987 3799847

Shulman KI: Clock-drawing: is it the ideal cognitive screening test? Int J Geriatr Psychiatry 15(6):548–561, 2000 10861923

Simon SS, Cordás TA, Bottino CM: Cognitive behavioral therapies in older adults with depression and cognitive deficits: a systematic review. Int J Geriatr Psychiatry 30(3):223–233, 2015 25521935

Sivertsen B, Omvik S, Pallesen S, et al: Cognitive behavioral therapy vs zopiclone for treatment of chronic primary insomnia in older adults: a randomized controlled trial. JAMA 295(24):2851–2858, 2006 16804151

Steffens DC, Blazer DG, Thakur ME (eds): The American Psychiatric Publishing Textbook of Geriatric Psychiatry, 5th Edition. Arlington, VA, American Psychiatric Publishing, 2015

Stoffers JM, Völlm BA, Rücker G, et al: Psychological therapies for people with borderline personality disorder. Cochrane Database Syst Rev 8:CD005652, 2012 22895952

Stroup TS, Gerhard T, Crystal S, et al: Comparative effectiveness of clozapine and standard antipsychotic treatment in adults with schizophrenia. Am J Psychiatry 173(2):166–173, 2016 26541815

Substance Abuse and Mental Health Services Administration: Family Psychoeducation: Building Your Program, HHS Publ No SMA-09-4422. Rockville, MD, Center for Mental Health Services, Substance Abuse and Mental Health Services Administration, 2009.

Substance Abuse and Mental Health Services Administration: Motivational interviewing. 2012. Available at: http://www.integration.samhsa.gov/clinical-practice/motivational-interviewing. Accessed August 18, 2016.

Substance Abuse and Mental Health Services Administration: Results From the 2013 National Survey on Drug Use and Health: Summary of National Findings (NSDUH Series H-48, HHS Publ No [SMA] 14-4863). Rockville, MD, Substance Abuse and Mental Health Services Administration, 2014. Available at: http://www.samhsa.gov/data/sites/default/files/NSDUHresultsPDFWHTML2013/Web/NSDUHresults2013.htm. Accessed August 18, 2016.

Substance Abuse and Mental Health Services Administration: Screening tools. 2015. Available at: http://www.integration.samhsa.gov/clinical-practice/screening-tools#suicide. Accessed August 18, 2016.

Suicide Prevention Resource Center: Patient safety plan template. 2015. Available at: http://www.sprc.org/sites/sprc.org/files/SafetyPlanTemplate.pdf. Accessed August 18, 2016.

Sun H, Palcza J, Card D, et al: Effects of suvorexant: an orexin receptor antagonist on respiration during sleep in patients with obstructive sleep apnea. J Clin Sleep Med 12(1)9–17, 2016

Sundsted KK, Burton MC, Shah R, Lapid MI: Preanesthesia medical evaluation for electroconvulsive therapy: a review of the literature. J ECT 30(1):35–42, 2014 24091900

Tannenbaum C, Martin P, Tamblyn R, et al: Reduction of inappropriate benzodiazepine prescriptions among older adults through direct patient education: the EMPOWER cluster randomized trial. JAMA Intern Med 174(6):890–898, 2014 24733354

Teri L, Logsdon RG, Uomoto J, McCurry SM: Behavioral treatment of depression in dementia patients: a controlled clinical trial. J Gerontol B Psychol Sci Soc Sci 52(4):159–166, 1997 9224439

Thakur ME, Blazer DG, Steffens DC (eds): Clinical Manual of Geriatric Psychiatry. Washington, DC, American Psychiatric Publishing, 2013

Tinetti ME: Performance-oriented assessment of mobility problems in elderly patients. J Am Geriatr Soc 34(2):119–126, 1986 3944402

Tinetti ME, Kumar C: The patient who falls: "It's always a trade-off." JAMA 303(3):258–266, 2010 20085954

Tomes N: Remaking the American Patient: How Madison Avenue and Modern Medicine Turned Patients Into Consumers. Chapel Hill, University of North Carolina Press, 2016

Tzimos A, Samokhvalov V, Kramer M, et al: Safety and tolerability of oral paliperidone extended-release tablets in elderly patients with schizophrenia: a double-blind, placebo-controlled study with six-month open-label extension. Am J Geriatr Psychiatry 16(1):31–43, 2008 18165460

Unützer J, Tang L, Oishi S, et al: Reducing suicidal ideation in depressed older primary care patients. J Am Geriatr Soc 54(10):1550–1556, 2006 17038073

Unützer J, Harbin H, Schoenbaum M, Druss B: The Collaborative Care Model: An Approach for Integrating Physical and Mental Health Care in Medicaid Health Homes. HEALTH HOME Information Resource Center Brief, May 2013. Available at: http://www.medicaid.gov/State-Resource-Center/Medicaid-State-Technical-Assistance/Health-Homes-Technical-Assistance/Downloads/HH-IRC-Collaborative-5-13.pdf. Accessed August 18, 2016.

U.S. Department of Health and Human Services: National Alzheimer's Project Act. August 3, 2016. Available at: https://aspe.hhs.gov/national-alzheimers-project-act. Accessed August 18, 2016.

U.S. Department of Veterans Affairs: Caregiver services. 2016. Available at: http://www.caregiver.va.gov/support. Accessed August 18, 2016.

U.S. Food and Drug Administration: FDA approves Viibryd to treat major depressive disorder (news release). January 21, 2011. Available at: http://www.fda.gov/NewsEvents/Newsroom/PressAnnouncements/ucm240642.htm. Accessed August 18, 2016.

U.S. Food and Drug Administration: FDA Drug Safety Communication: FDA reporting mental health drug ziprasidone (Geodon) associated with rare but potentiall fatal skin reactions, 2014a. Available at: http://www.fda.gov/Drugs/DrugSafety/ucm426391.htm. Accessed August 27, 2016.

U.S. Food and Drug Administration: Questions and Answers: Risk of next-morning impairment after use of insomnia drugs; FDA requires lower recommended doses for certain drugs containing zolpidem (Ambien, Ambien CR, Edluar, and Zolpimist), 2014b.

Available at: http://www.fda.gov/Drugs/DrugSafety/ucm334041.htm. Accessed August 18, 2016.

U.S. Food and Drug Administration: FDA Drug Safety Communication: FDA approves new label changes and dosing for zolpidem products and a recommendation to avoid driving the day after using Ambien CR. January 15, 2016. Available at: http://www.fda.gov/drugs/drugsafety/ucm352085.htm. Accessed August 18, 2016.

Vaccarino AL, Sills T, Anderson KE, et al: Assessment of depression, anxiety and apathy in prodromal and early Huntington disease. PLoS Curr Jun 17; 3:RRN1242, 2011

van Reekum R, Stuss DT, Ostrander L: Apathy: why care? J Neuropsychiatry Clin Neurosci 17(1):7–19, 2005 15746478

Verwijk E, Comijs HC, Kok RM, et al: Neurocognitive effects after brief pulse and ultrabrief pulse unilateral electroconvulsive therapy for major depression: a review. J Affect Disord 140(3):233–243, 2012 22595374

Vigen CLP, Mack WJ, Keefe RSE, et al: Cognitive effects of atypical antipsychotic medications in patients with Alzheimer's disease: outcomes from CATIE-AD. Am J Psychiatry 168(8):831–839, 2011 21572163

Viswanathan M, Golin, CE, Jones CD, et al: Interventions to improve adherence to self-administered medications for chronic diseases in the United States: a systematic review. Ann Intern Med 157(11):785–795, 2012 22964778

Wang S, Blazer DG: Depression and cognition in the elderly. Annu Rev Clin Psychol 11:331–360, 2015 25581234

Weintraub D, Koester J, Potenza MN, et al: Impulse control disorders in Parkinson disease: a cross-sectional study of 3090 patients. Arch Neurol 67(5):589–595, 2010 20457959

Winkelman JW: Insomnia disorder. N Engl J Med 373(15):1437–1444, 2015 26444730

Woolcott JC, Richardson KJ, Wiens MO, et al: Meta-analysis of the impact of 9 medication classses on falls in eldery persons. Arch Intern Med 169(21):1952–1960, 2009 19933955

World Health Organization: Measuring Health and Disability: Manual for WHO Disability Assessment Schedule (WHODAS 2.0). Edited by Üstün TB, Kostanjsek N, Chatterji S, et al. Geneva, World Health Organization, 2010

Yesavage JA, Brink TL, Rose TL, et al: Development and validation of a geriatric depression screening scale: a preliminary report. J Psychiatr Res 17(1):37–49, 1982–1983 7183759

Zohar J, Nutt DJ, Kupfer DJ, et al: A proposal for an updated neuropsychopharmacological nomenclature. Eur Neuropsychopharmacol 24(7):1004–1015, 2014 24630385

Page numbers printed in **boldface** type refer to tables or figures.

Antidepressants *(continued)*
    response of depressed older
        patients to first-line, 75
    substance-induced mania
        and, 57
Antihistamines, 35
Antipsychotics
    geriatric-appropriate doses of
        for schizophrenia, 60
    psychopharmacology for
        psychotic disorders and,
        291, **292–295,** 296–297
Antisocial personality disorder,
    177, 181
Anxiety. *See also* Anxiety
        disorders
    alcohol withdrawal and, 144
    cannabis withdrawal and,
        148
    illness anxiety disorder and,
        120
    sedative, hypnotic, or
        anxiolytic withdrawal
        and, 160
    somatic symptom disorder
        and, 119
    tobacco use disorder and, 166
Anxiety disorders
    differential diagnosis of
        obsessive-compulsive
        disorder and, 112
    DSM-5 diagnostic criteria for,
        193–194
    prevalence of in older adults,
        8
    psychopharmacology for,
        296–297, **298–300, 305**
    30-Minute Older Adult
        Diagnostic Interview
        and, 87, 106–110
Apathy, and major
    neurocognitive disorder,
    46–47
Aphoria, and thought process,
    211
Appearance
    histrionic personality
        disorder and, 183

mental status examination
    and, 209
Appetite
    cannabis intoxication and, 148
    cannabis withdrawal and, 148
    stimulant withdrawal and,
        164
    tobacco use disorder and, 166
Aripiprazole, **292**
Asenapine, **292**
Association for Frontotemporal
    Degeneration, 248
Ataque de nervios, 219, 229
Atrial fibrillation, and panic
    attacks, 25
Attention-seeking, and
    histrionic personality
    disorder, 177–178, 183
Avoidance
    borderline personality
        disorder and, 182
    specific phobia and, 106
Avoidant personality disorder,
    178, 184–185
Avoidant/restrictive food intake
    disorder, 122–124

Backup proxy, for primary
    caregiver, 15
Barthel Index of Activities of
    Daily Living, **253**
Behavior. *See also* Aggression;
    Agitation; Criminal behav-
    ior; Distractibility; Eccentric
    behavior; Help seeking;
    Impulsivity; Irritability
    apathy in major
        neurocognitive disorder
        and, 46–47
    assessment of, 255–257
    common examples of distress
        and, 6
    help rejection and, 74–75
    histrionic personality
        disorder and seductive,
        183
    illness anxiety disorder and,
        120

intermittent explosive
disorder and, 139
mental status examination
and, 209–210
nonpharmacological inter-
ventions and, 245–247
Benzodiazepines, 296–297, 301–
302
Bereavement, and depression,
41–42. *See also* Grief
Berg Balance Scale, **254**
Best practices, and treatment
planning, 320–321
Bipolar and related disorders
depression and, 46
DSM-5 diagnostic criteria for,
191–192
prevalence of in older adults,
8
psychopharmacology for,
286, **287–290**, 291, **303**
30-Minute Older Adult
Diagnostic Interview
and, 98–103
Body dysmorphic disorder, 111–
112
Body-focused repetitive
behaviors, 113
Body mass index (BMI),
antipsychotics and
monitoring of, 296
Borderline personality disorder,
177, 181–182
Brain stimulation therapies. *See*
Deep brain stimulation;
Electroconvulsive therapy;
Transcranial magnetic
stimulation; Vagal nerve
stimulation
failure to respond to other
interventions and, 309
need for clinical research
trials on, 314
Breathing-related sleep
disorders, diagnosis of, 49–
50. *See also* Sleep apnea;
Sleep-related
hypoventilation

Brief Psychiatric Rating Scale
(BPRS), **232**
Brief psychotic disorder, 97–98
Bulimia nervosa, 122, **198**
Bupropion, **283**
Burnout, of caregivers, 14
Buspirone, 297, **298**

Caffeine intoxication, 57, 144–
145
Caffeine withdrawal, 145–146
Cannabis intoxication, 148
Cannabis use disorder, 146–147
Cannabis withdrawal, 148–149
Capgras delusions, 61
Carbamazepine, 286, **287**, **290**
Cardiac arrhythmia, and
caffeine intoxication, 145
Cardiovascular complications,
of electroconvulsive
therapy, 310–311
Caregivers
concepts defining geriatric
psychiatry and care for, 6
management of self-neglect,
self-harm, and suicidal
behavior, 67
psychoeducation classes for,
243–245
respite programs for, 258–259
stepwise approach to
differential diagnosis
and conflicts with, 204
support groups for, 14, 247
therapeutic alliance and, 13–
15
treatment planning and goals
of, 319–320
use of term, viii
Case example
of aggression and agitation,
64
of bereavement, 41
of breathing-related sleep
disorder, 49, 50
of deep brain stimulation, 312
of delirium, 32–33, 55–57
of delusional disorder, 61

Discontinuation, of medications, **303–304,** 306

Disease, definition of, 229, 316

Disease/disorder-based model, of treatment planning, 27

Disruptive, impulse-control, and conduct disorders, and 30-Minute Older Adult Diagnostic Interview, 138–140

Dissociation. *See also* Dissociative disorders

borderline personality disorder and, 182

30-Minute Older Adult Diagnostic Interview and, 87

Dissociative amnesia, 116–117

Dissociative disorders, and 30-Minute Older Adult Diagnostic Interview, 116–118

Dissociative identity disorder, 117

Distractibility

bipolar disorder and, 99, 101

mental status examination and, 211

Diuresis, and caffeine intoxication, 145

Divalproex, **288**

Dizziness

inhalant intoxication and, 153

panic disorder and, 108

Doses and dosing, and medications

golden rule of for older adults, 274, 285

noncompliance and intentional skipping of, **277**

Doxepin, 297, **298**

Dreams. *See also* Nightmare disorder

posttraumatic stress disorder and, 114

stimulant withdrawal and, 164

Drowsiness, and caffeine withdrawal, 145

Drug(s), and diagnosis of common disorders in older adults, **32,** 35. *See also* Medications

Drug-drug interactions, and polypharmacy, 301

Dry mouth, and cannabis intoxication, 148

DSM-IV-TR

conditions coded on Axis IV of, 187

criteria for depressive disorders and, 41, 43

DSM-5. *See also* Cultural Formulation Interview; 15-Minute Older Adult Diagnostic Interview; Level I and Level II Cross-Cutting Symptom Measures; Level of Personality Functioning Scale; 30-Minute Older Adult Diagnostic Interview; World Health Organization Disability Assessment Schedule 2.0

assessment tools for brief interviews in, 20

bereavement delay and diagnosis of major depressive disorder, 43

categorical model of mental illness in, 213

as consensus manual developed by experts, 324

confirming diagnosis using criteria in, 21–23

definition of mental disorder in, 207

diagnostic criteria for

anorexia nervosa, **198**

bipolar I disorder, **191**

bipolar II disorder, **192**

bulimia nervosa, **198**

conversion disorder, **197**

delirium, **33–34, 199**

generalized anxiety disorder, **194**

15-Minute Older Adult
Diagnostic Interview
and, 70
major neurocognitive
disorder and, 39–40

Gabapentin, **298**
GAD-7. *See* Generalized Anxiety
Disorder 7-item Scale
Gait, assessment of, 26, 252, **254,**
255
Gambling disorder, 169–170
Gastrointestinal disturbance,
and caffeine intoxication,
145
Gender dysphoria, and 30-
Minute Older Adult
Diagnostic Interview, 137–
138
Generalized anxiety disorder
cognitive-behavioral therapy
for, 268
DSM-5 diagnostic criteria for,
194
30-Minute Older Adult
Diagnostic Interview
and, 109–110
Generalized Anxiety Disorder 7-
item Scale (GAD-7), 17, 69
Genito-pelvic pain/penetration
disorder, 134
Geriatric Depression Scale
(GDS), 46, **231**
Geriatric psychiatry, 5–6
Gerontological Environmental
Modifications Assessment,
255
Geropsychologists, and neuro-
psychology reports, 257
Get-up and Go Test, **254**
Global mental status, and rating
scales, **232**
Goal-directed activity, and
bipolar disorder, 99, 101
Grandiosity
bipolar disorder and, 99, 101
narcissistic personality
disorder and, 183

Grief. *See also* Bereavement
debate on boundaries
between mental illness
and normal age-related
changes, vii
diagnosis of major depressive
episode and, 45
Guidelines
for clinical practice by
American Psychiatric
Association, 320–321
for sleep hygiene, **49**
for 30-Minute Older Adult
Diagnostic Interview,
83–84
Guilt, and major depressive
disorder, 104

Hallucinations
alcohol withdrawal and, 144
mental status examination
and, 212
schizophrenia and, 96
sedative, hypnotic, or
anxiolytic withdrawal
and, 160
Haloperidol, **293**
Headache, and caffeine
withdrawal, 145
Health care. *See also* Medical
conditions; Palliative care;
Physicians
integration of with mental
health care, 28–29, 62–63
problem of uncoordinated
care for older adults, 3–4
Health insurance, and case
management, 258
Healthy Aging Brain Medical
Home, 29
Help seeking, cultural factors in,
220–221
Histrionic personality disorder,
178, 182–183
HIV infection, and delirium, 175
Hoarding disorder, 112
Holmes-Rahe Stress Scale, 41
Home care services, 258, 259

National Institute of Health, and Senior Health web site, 262
National Institute of Mental Health, 234, 249, 285
Nausea
    alcohol withdrawal and, 144
    opioid withdrawal and, 157
    panic disorder and, 108
    sedative, hypnotic, or anxiolytic withdrawal and, 160
    stimulant intoxication and, 163
Neglect, and elder abuse, 263. *See also* Self-neglect
Neologisms, and thought process, 211
Nervousness
    caffeine intoxication and, 144
    cannabis withdrawal and, 148
Neurocognitive disorders. *See also* Major neurocognitive disorder; Mild neurocognitive disorder
    diagnosis of, 36–41
    DSM-5 criteria for, **198**
    medical or neurological disorders as risk factors for, 24–25
    rating scales for, **231**
    30-Minute Older Adult Diagnostic Interview and, 170–176
Neurological disorders
    differential diagnosis and, 24–27
    mania or psychotic symptoms and, 57, 59
Neuropsychiatric Inventory (NPI), **231**
Neuropsychological testing, of cognition and behavior, 255–257
NeuroStar TMS Therapy system, 312
Nightmare disorder, 130
NIH Senior Health, 249

Noncompliance with psychopharmacology, 274, 276, **277,** 278
Non-rapid eye movement sleep arousal disorder, 130
Normality, boundaries between abnormality and, 207
Nortriptyline, **282**
Nutritional deficiency, and avoidant/restrictive food intake disorder, 123

Obsessions
    mental status examination and, 212
    30-Minute Older Adult Diagnostic Interview and, 87, 111
Obsessive-compulsive disorder
    DSM-5 criteria for, **194**
    prevalence of in older adults, 8
    30-Minute Older Adult Diagnostic Interview and, 110–112
Obsessive-compulsive personality disorder, 178, 186–187
Obstructive sleep apnea hypopnea (OSA). *See also* Sleep apnea
    diagnosis of, 49–51
    30-Minute Older Adult Diagnostic Interview and, 128–129
Olanzapine, **293**
Older adults. *See also* Age and aging; Patients; *specific disorders*
    changing definition of, 5
    customization of psychoeducational interventions for, 244
    importance of psychotherapy as treatment option for, 265
    living options for, 251–252
    mobile apps for, 247

onset of mania in, 57
prevalence of mental
    disorders in, 7–8
problem of uncoordinated
    medical care for, 3–4
rapid growth in population
    of, 324
as sexually active, 63
skills for care of, 4–5
suicide rates for, 77
Open-ended questions, and
    therapeutic alliance, 12
Opioid intoxication, 156
Opioid use disorder, 154–156
Opioid withdrawal, 156–157
Oppositional defiant disorder,
    140
OSA. *See* Obstructive sleep
    apnea
Other specified diagnosis, and
    differential diagnosis, 207
Other (or unknown) substance
    use disorder, 167–168
Other (or unknown) substance
    withdrawal, 169
Over-the-counter medications,
    and cognitive impairment,
    35

PACE programs, 259
Paliperidone, **294**
Palliative care, and management
    of self-neglect, self-harm,
    and suicidal behavior, 67
Palliative Performance Scale, **253**
Palpitations, and phencyclidine
    or other hallucinogen use
    disorder, 151
Panic attacks, 107, 108–109, 229
Panic disorder
    DSM-5 diagnostic criteria for,
        193–194
    30-Minute Older Adult
        Diagnostic Interview
        and, 107–109
Paranoia. *See also* Suspicion
    borderline personality
        disorder and, 182

schizotypal personality
    disorder and, 180
Paranoid personality disorder,
    177, 178–179
Paresthesias, and panic disorder,
    108
Parkinson's disease, 24, 27, 59,
    176
Paroxetine, **280**
Patient(s). *See also* Older adults;
    Patient history; Therapeutic
    alliance
    treatment planning and goals
        of, 319–320
    use of term, viii
    views of disease and illness
        by, 229, 316
Patient Health Questionnaire 9-
    item depression scale
    (PHQ-9), 17, 18–19, 37, 39,
    69, **232**
Patient history, and 15-Minute
    Older Adult Diagnostic
    Interview, 72–74
Performance-Oriented
    Assessment of Balance, **254**
Performance-Oriented
    Assessment of Gait, **254**
Periodic limb movement
    disorder (PLMD), 50–51,
    52–53
Perphenazine, **294**
Persecutory delusions, in older
    adults without dementia, 61
Persistent complex bereavement
    disorder, 42
Persistent depressive disorder,
    193
Personality change due to
    another medical condition,
    187
Personality disorders, and 30-
    Minute Older Adult Diag-
    nostic Interview, 177–187
Personality traits
    Level of Personality
        Functioning Scale and,
        221–222

Personality traits *(continued)*
    30-Minute Older Adult Diagnostic Interview and, 88
Phantom boarder syndrome, 61
Phencyclidine or other hallucinogen use disorder, 149–151
Phenobarbital, **290**
Phenytoin, **290**
Phobia, and mental status examination, 212. *See also* Specific phobia
PHQ-9. *See* Patient Health Questionnaire 9-item depression scale
Physical impairment, and noncompliance with medications, **277**
Physiological reactions, and posttraumatic stress disorder, 114
Pica, 123
Placebo effect, and medication noncompliance, 278
Planning. *See* Treatment
PLMD. *See* Periodic limb movement disorder
Pocket Guide to the DSM-5 Diagnostic Exam (Nussbaum 2013), 83
Polypharmacy, 297, 301–302, **303–305**, 306
Polysomnography, 127, 129
Positive aging, and schizophrenia, 59–60
Posttraumatic stress disorder (PTSD)
    DSM-5 criteria for, **195–196**
    prevalence of in older adults, 8
    30-Minute Older Adult Diagnostic Interview and, 113–116
Premature ejaculation, 133
Preoccupation
    dependent personality disorder and, 185

narcissistic personality disorder and, 183
paranoid personality disorder and, 178
illness anxiety disorder and, 120
Prevalence
    of apathy in Alzheimer's disease, 47
    of comorbidity of mental disorders, 23
    of delusions in older adults, 61
    of mental disorders in older adults, 7–8
Prevention of Suicide in Primary Care Elderly: Collaborative Trial (PROSPECT), 28
Primidone, **290**
Prion disease, and delirium, 175
Problem lists, and treatment planning, 315–318
Problem-solving therapy, **266,** 270–271
PST. *See* Problem-solving therapy
PST for executive dysfunction and problem-adaptation therapy (PATH), 271
Psychiatric history, and 30-Minute Older Adult Diagnostic Interview, 85–86
Psychodynamic psychotherapy, **266,** 267–268
Psychoeducation
    classes in, 243–245
    web resources for, 248–249
Psychology. *See also* Geropsychologists; Psychosocial interventions
    factors in medication noncompliance and, 278
    self-harm or self-neglect and, 67
Psychomotor agitation or retardation
    alcohol withdrawal and, 144
    caffeine intoxication and, 145

Selegiline, **283**

Self-awareness, and characteristics of mental distress versus mental illness, 7

Self-direction, and Level of Personality Functioning Scale, **223–227**

Self-esteem
bipolar disorder and, 99, 101
diagnosis of grief versus major depressive episode and, 45

Self-harm, and diagnosis of mental disorders in older adults, 64–67

Self-image
anorexia nervosa and, 122
posttraumatic stress disorder and, 114

Self-neglect, and self-harm, 67

Self-resolution, and mental distress, 7

Separation anxiety disorder, 107

Sequenced Treatment Alternatives to Relieve Depression (STAR*D) trial, 285

Serotonin-norepinephrine reuptake inhibitors (SNRIs), 279, **281–282,** 285

Sertraline, 279, **280**

Severity, and rating scales, 230, 234

Sexual dysfunction
diagnosis of, 63
15-Minute Older Adult Diagnostic Interview and, 75–76
30-Minute Older Adult Diagnostic Interview and, 131–137

Short Confusion Assessment Method (Short CAM), 33

Short Michigan Alcoholism Screening Test—Geriatric Version (SMAST-G), **233**

Short-term supportive interventions, mental distress and response to, 7

Skilled nursing facilities, and long-term-care planning, 261

Sleep, disturbances of. *See also* Insomnia; Sleep-wake disorders
bipolar disorder and, 99, 101
cannabis withdrawal and, 148
diagnosis of disrupted in older adults, 47–51
generalized anxiety disorder and, 109
posttraumatic stress disorder and, 115

Sleep apnea, and cognitive impairment, 36. *See also* Obstructive sleep apnea hypopnea

Sleep diary, 48

Sleep hygiene, **49**

Sleep-related hallucinations, 60

Sleep-related hypoventilation, 129

Sleep-wake disorders. *See also* Insomnia; Sleep
DSM-5 criteria for, **198**
psychopharmacology for, 296–297, **298–300, 305**
30-Minute Older Adult Diagnostic Interview and, 87–88, 124–131

Social anxiety, and schizotypal personality disorder, 180

Social anxiety disorder, 107

Social history, and 30-Minute Older Adult Diagnostic Interview, 88–89. *See also* Interpersonal relationships

Somatic symptom and related disorders
cannabis withdrawal and, 149
depression and, 46
DSM-5 criteria for, **197**
psychological factors affecting medication conditions and, 62

Treatment. *See also* Brain stimulation therapies; Mental
health care; Psychoeduca-
tion; Psychopharmacology;
Psychosocial interventions;
Psychotherapy; Treatment
planning
functional benefit of, 5–6
nonpharmacological
interventions for
cognitive and behavioral
difficulties, 245–247
therapeutic alliance as key to
successful, 9–12
Treatment planning
best practices for, 320–321
care coordination and, 27–28
patient and caregiver goals,
319–320
problem lists and, 315–318
steps in for older adults, **321**
Tremor
alcohol withdrawal and, 144
functional assessment and, 27
Trichotillomania, 113
Tricyclic antidepressants, 279,
282, 301

U.S. Centers for Medicare &
Medicaid Services, 234
U.S. National Alzheimer's
Project Act (2012), 323
Unspecified diagnosis, and
differential diagnosis, 207
Upper extremity examination,
and neurological
examination, 26–27
UpToDate (web site), 249
Urine toxicology screens, 276

Vagal nerve stimulation (VNS),
313–314
Valproic acid, 286, **288, 290,** 301
Vascular disease, and delirium,
175
Venlafaxine, **282**
Verbigeration, and thought
process, 211

Veterans, and respite services,
258–259
Vilazodone, **284**
Vision, and visual impairment.
See also Eye contact
hallucinations due to, 60
inhalant intoxication and, 154
phencyclidine or other
hallucinogen use
disorder and blurring of,
151
Visual hallucinations, due to
visual impairment, 60
Vortioxetine, **284**

Web sites. *See* Internet
Weight loss or gain
anorexia nervosa and, 122
avoidant/restrictive food
intake disorder and, 123
cannabis withdrawal and,
148
major depressive disorder
and, 104
WHODAS 2.0. *See* World Health
Organization Disability
Schedule 2.0
Withdrawal
alcohol use disorder and, 142
opioid use disorder and, 155
sedative, hypnotic, or
anxiolytic use disorder
and, 158–159
tobacco use disorder and, 165
World Health Organization, 234.
See also ICD-10-CM codes
World Health Organization
Disability Assessment
Schedule 2.0, 221
Word salad, 211

Yawning, and opioid
withdrawal, 157

Zaleplon, **299**
Z drugs, 297
Ziprasidone, **295**
Zolpidem, **300,** 301